NEW ZEALAND

calorie counter

PENGUIN BOOKS

PENGUIN BOOKS
Published by the Penguin Group
Penguin Group (NZ), 67 Apollo Drive, Rosedale,
Auckland 0632, New Zealand (a division of Penguin New Zealand Pty Ltd)
Penguin Group (USA) Inc., 375 Hudson Street,
New York, New York 10014, USA
Penguin Group (Canada), 90 Eglinton Avenue East, Suite 700, Toronto,
Ontario, M4P 2Y3, Canada (a division of Penguin Canada Books Inc.)
Penguin Books Ltd, 80 Strand, London, WC2R 0RL, England
Penguin Ireland, 25 St Stephen's Green,
Dublin 2, Ireland (a division of Penguin Books Ltd)
Penguin Group (Australia), 707 Collins Street, Melbourne,
Victoria 3008, Australia (a division of Penguin Australia Pty Ltd)
Penguin Books India Pvt Ltd, 11, Community Centre,
Panchsheel Park, New Delhi – 110 017, India
Penguin Books (South Africa) (Pty) Ltd, Block D, Rosebank Office Park,
181 Jan Smuts Avenue, Parktown North, Gauteng 2193, South Africa
Penguin (Beijing) Ltd, 7F, Tower B, Jiaming Center, 27 East Third Ring Road North,
Chaoyang District, Beijing 100020, China

Penguin Books Ltd, Registered Offices: 80 Strand, London, WC2R 0RL, England

First published by Whitcoulls Publishers, 1974
First published by Penguin Group (NZ) Ltd, 1988, revised and updated
2006 (reprinted five times), 2009 (reprinted four times),
2011, 2013, 2015
1 3 5 7 9 10 8 6 4 2

Copyright © Penguin Group (NZ), 1988, 2015

The right of Penguin Group (NZ) to be identified as the author of this work in terms of
section 96 of the Copyright Act 1994 is hereby asserted.

Designed and typeset by Sarah Healey, © Penguin Group (NZ)
Weight Control Made Easy text by Anna Sloan
Cover image from www.iStockphoto.com
Printed and bound in Australia by Griffin Press,
an Accredited ISO AS/NZS 14001 Environmental Management Systems Printer

ISBN 978-0-143-57207-7

A catalogue record for this book is available
from the National Library of New Zealand.

www.penguin.co.nz

Products have been included only where accurate information could be obtained.

CONTENTS

WEIGHT CONTROL MADE EASY

Every day we seem to be bombarded with new diets and weight-loss regimes. But most nutrition experts agree that in order to lose weight, energy eaten should be less than energy expended. In this book you will find the calorie and kilojoule values of a wide range of New Zealand foods and drinks to help you understand how much energy the foods you eat are giving you. By substituting foods and drinks that are lower in calories/kilojoules you will find you can easily control your weight and still enjoy a varied and interesting diet.

You will soon remember which foods are better for you than others. The healthy heart diagram (see page 8) is a good reminder of which major food groups contribute to a healthy diet and the healthy plate model (see page 9) is an easy way to ensure you eat the correct proportions of different foods for a healthy weight.

WHAT IS A CALORIE/KILOJOULE?

A calorie is the unit used for stating the energy value of a food and also the energy requirement of an individual. Foods with many calories can give us excess energy; foods with fewer calories provide lower energy.

Kilojoule is the metric term for a unit of calorie (1 calorie = 4.2 kilojoules). Both units are used in this counter. Note that due to rounding in the calculations, you will find slight variations in the calorie/kilojoule ratios in this book.

USE YOUR COUNTER EVERY DAY

Keeping an eye on what goes into your body is the first step to weight loss. Often we forget about or disregard the snacks or drinks that we consume and these small things add up. If you only want to lose a few kilograms, start by keeping a record of what you eat in a day, then use this book to analyse the calorie/kilojoule content of your daily food intake. Eat more lower-rated foods (such as green vegetables, salads and fresh fruit) than higher-rated ones. The healthy plate model on page 9 provides a straight-forward visual guideline to help you remember this.

If your weight reduction requirement is more serious, look on pages 10–12 for the ideal calorie/kilojoule intake for your height. The recommended intakes are based on a BMI (Body Mass Index) of 23. This is the mid-point of the healthy weight for height options (see the Healthy Weight Range for Men & Women table on page 9). Use this book to plan your daily menus, checking that they keep within the appropriate calorie/ kilojoule allocation.

With the *Calorie Counter*, you get to choose your own foods – foods that you enjoy, that fit with your lifestyle and budget, but enable you to achieve your weight reduction goal.

Start out slowly, perhaps by substituting a usual food or drink for a lower-calorie version. Shop around; eating well doesn't have to be expensive, but keep in mind that some cheaper versions of foods have higher calorie/kilojoule values than others. Whatever you do, DO NOT skip meals, especially breakfast. This will only make you hungrier and result in snacking on foods that might satisfy your immediate hunger, but may be higher in calories. Skipping meals also slows your metabolism, making the food you eat later in the day more likely to be stored as fat.

Make sure you don't cut out whole food groups; this may result in nutrient deficiencies or rapid weight loss that is too easily regained (with more!) when you stop 'dieting'.

HOW YOU CAN GAIN & LOSE WEIGHT

The energy produced by the calories/kilojoules you consume is released into and used by your body for all its activities. If you eat more than your system can burn up, the excess from all food groups becomes fat. Extra weight you may be carrying represents unused, stored energy.

You lose weight when you expend more energy than what you take in from the food you eat and therefore draw on the reserve calories/ kilojoules stored in your surplus fat. But it is seldom sufficient just to increase your physical activity. It takes a lot of exercise to burn up those surplus fat stores.

The real answer to efficient and long-lasting weight reduction is to reduce your daily intake of calories/kilojoules by consuming balanced, nutritious meals in combination with moderate daily exercise, over a longer period of time.

If you have a lot of weight to lose, you may experience a plateau. This is a period of at least three months where you no longer seem to lose weight despite eating carefully. Celebrate, as this is your body getting used to a new, lower weight. Continue with the healthy eating changes you have made, then revisit the steps above; stepping off the plateau into further weight reduction often requires only minor tweaking.

LOSING WEIGHT BY COUNTING CALORIES/KILOJOULES

Your personal daily requirement of calories/kilojoules to ensure a loss of weight of around 500g a week (on average) can be calculated the following way:

1. Look at the height/weight chart on page 9. Does your weight fit into the healthy range for your height? If it is over, or at the higher end of the scale, you might want to lose a few kilos.

2. Use the chart on pages 10–12 to find your daily calorie/kilojoule requirement for your height and level of exercise. Once you know what that is you can use this book to add up your calorie/kilojoule intake and see if you are meeting your requirements.

3. To lose weight, aim to reduce your intake by around 400–500kcals (1680–2095kj)/day. This should result in a weight loss of around 500–900g a week. It may be more initially as your eating habits change.

Losing more than 1kg a week may mean you are being overly restrictive. Slower weight loss of around 500–900g/week is more likely to be long-term weight loss. While a loss of between 500g and 900g a week may not seem very much, it does in effect mean a loss of 6–12kg in only three months, safely and with a minimum of hardship.

It is unwise and can be dangerous to reduce your intake below 1000 calories/4190 kilojoules a day. Very low-calorie diets may result in considerable loss of muscle tissue and fluid, which appears to be rapid weight loss, but is replaced very quickly when a more liberal diet is resumed. You are unlikely to meet your nutritional requirements if you are consuming less than 1000kcals/4190kj a day. Rapid weight loss also results in fatigue and irritability and can cause skin to wrinkle.

You should always see your doctor before starting a major weight-reduction campaign. They will, if necessary, help you to set realistic weight-reduction goals, taking into account your medical history, as well as your age, build and occupation. A ten percent weight loss should be enough to significantly improve most weight-related health conditions.

ESSENTIAL FOODS FOR GOOD HEALTH

The healthy heart diagram overleaf is a good way to show which foods should be eaten often and which foods should only be eaten occasionally or in small amounts. The layers represent major food groups that contribute to a healthy diet.

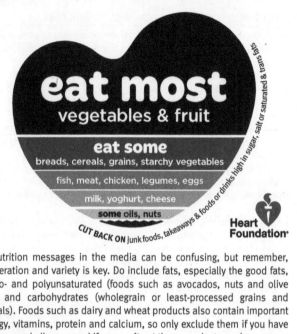

Nutrition messages in the media can be confusing, but remember, moderation and variety is key. Do include fats, especially the good fats, mono- and polyunsaturated (foods such as avocados, nuts and olive oils) and carbohydrates (wholegrain or least-processed grains and cereals). Foods such as dairy and wheat products also contain important energy, vitamins, protein and calcium, so only exclude them if you have a diagnosed allergy – and if you can't eat these products, make sure you include a suitable alternative.

USING THE HEALTHY PLATE MODEL

When planning or serving a meal, always try to ensure it is made up of at least half a plate of vegetables, a quarter of a plate (or a palm-size serving) of protein foods and a quarter (or a palm-size serving) of carbohydrate. You should have more carbohydrate in the day than protein serves, so at lunch you might have two serves (e.g. 2 slices of bread). Following this ratio guideline at lunch and dinner means you will be eating a nutritionally balanced, energy-appropriate meal. This helps to make you feel full, meaning you're less likely to choose higher-energy treat foods later in the day. Use this book to fill your plate with foods you love that meet your calorie/kilojoule goal!

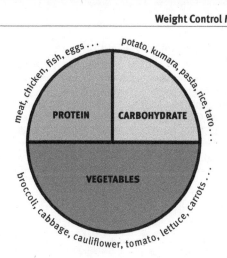

MAINTAINING YOUR NEW WEIGHT

Well done if you have achieved your target weight reduction. You may now be able to increase your daily calorie/kilojoule intake, especially if you remain active. Use the tables to check your new ideal calorie intake. Remember that maintaining healthy eating habits is the key to keeping weight off, so don't be tempted to go back to your old eating habits – save that higher-calorie/kilojoule food for special occasions. A treat is not a treat if you have it every day, so keep an eye on things and take action should your weight start to increase again.

HEALTHY WEIGHT RANGE FOR MEN & WOMEN

Measured in Height (cm) & Weight (kg)							
142	40–50	155	48–60	168	56–71	180	65–81
145	42–52	157	50–62	170	58–72	183	68–85
147	44–55	160	51–64	173	60–75	185	69–86
150	45–56	163	53–66	175	62–77	188	71–88
152	46–58	165	55–68	178	63–79	190	72–90

DAILY MAINTENANCE CALORIE/KILOJOULE ALLOWANCE

It is very difficult to say exactly how many calories/kilojoules any one person should be consuming each day. However, here are some basic guidelines, based on height and movement frequency, that should give you a good idea of how many calories/kilojoules you should be eating as part of a healthy diet. These tables are separated by how active a person is: inactive (i.e. work in an office, drive/bus to work), moderately active (on your feet for four–five hours/day) and very active (on your feet all day, plus exercising). Obviously, the more active you are, the more calories/kilojoules you can consume because your body is using the extra energy.

Age 18–30 years							
Men				Women			
Height	Inactive	Moderate	Active	Height	Inactive	Moderate	Active
cm	cal/kj	cal/kj	cal/kj	cm	cal/kj	cal/kj	cal/kj
142	1655/6953	1931/8112	2759/11588	142	1397/5866	1629/6843	2328/9776
146	1709/7180	1994/8376	2849/11966	146	1450/6089	169/7104	2416/10148
150	1763/7406	2057/8641	2939/12344	150	1503/6312	1753/7364	2505/10520
154	1817/7633	2120/8905	3029/12722	154	1556/6535	1815/7624	2593/10892
158	1853/7784	2162/9082	3089/12974	158	1591/6684	1857/7798	2652/11140
162	1907/8011	2225/9346	3179/13352	162	1645/6907	1919/8058	2741/11512
166	1961/8238	2288/9611	3269/13730	166	1698/7130	1981/8319	2830/11884
170	2015/8465	2351/9876	3359/14108	170	1751/7354	2043/8579	2918/12256
174	2087/8767	2435/10228	3479/14612	174	1822/7651	2125/8926	3036/12752
178	2141/8994	2498/10493	3569/15368	178	1875/7874	2187/9187	3125/13124
182	2195/9221	2561/10758	3659/15368	182	1928/8098	2249/9447	3213/13496
186	2267/9523	2645/11110	3779/15872	186	1999/8395	2332/9794	3331/13992
190	2321/9750	2708/11375	3869/16250	190	2052/8618	2394/10055	3420/14364
194	2393/10052	2792/11728	3989/16754	194	2123/8916	2477/10402	3538/14860
198	2447/10279	2855/11992	4079/17132	198	2176/9139	2539/10662	3627/15232
202	2519/10582	2939/12345	4199/17636	202	2247/9437	2621/11010	3745/15728

Age 30–60 years							
Men				Women			
Height	Inactive	Moderate	Active	Height	Inactive	Moderate	Active
cm	cal/kj	cal/kj	cal/kj	cm	cal/kj	cal/kj	cal/kj
142	1675/7033	1954/8205	2791/11722	142	1458/6122	1701/7143	2430/10204
146	1716/7206	2002/8407	2860/12010	146	1487/6245	1735/7286	2478/10408
150	1757/7379	2050/8609	2928/12298	150	1516/6367	1769/7428	2527/10612
154	1798/7552	2098/8810	2997/12586	154	1545/6490	1803/7571	2575/10816
158	1825/7667	2130/8945	3042/12778	158	1565/6571	1825/7666	2608/10952
162	1867/7840	2178/9146	3111/13066	162	1594/6694	1859/7809	2656/11156
166	1908/8012	2226/9348	3180/13354	166	1623/6816	1893/7952	2705/11360
170	1949/8185	2274/9549	3248/13642	170	1652/6938	1927/8095	2753/11564
174	2004/8416	2338/9818	3340/14026	174	1691/7102	1973/8285	2818/11836
178	2045/8588	2386/10020	3408/14314	178	1720/7224	2007/8428	2867/12040
182	2086/8761	2434/10221	3477/14602	182	1749/7346	2041/8571	2915/12244
186	2141/8992	2498/10490	3568/14986	186	1788/7510	2086/8761	2980/12516
190	2182/9164	2546/10962	3637/15274	190	1817/7632	2120/8904	3029/12720
194	2237/9395	2610/10961	3728/15658	194	1856/7795	2165/9094	3093/12992
198	2278/9568	2685/11162	3797/15946	198	1885/7918	2199/9237	3142/13196
202	2333/9798	2722/11431	3888/16330	202	1924/8081	2245/9428	3207/13468

Age 60+ years (continued over page)							
Men				Women			
Height	Inactive	Moderate	Active	Height	Inactive	Moderate	Active
cm	cal/kj	cal/kj	cal/kj	cm	cal/kj	cal/kj	cal/kj
142	1347/5656	1571/6598	2244/9428	142	1287/5404	1501/6304	2144/9006

| Age 60+ years continued . . . | | | | | | | |
| Men | | | Women | | | | |
Height	Inactive	Moderate	Active	Height	Inactive	Moderate	Active
146	1389/5832	1620/6804	2314/9720	146	1319/5540	1539/6464	2199/9234
150	1431/6008	1669/7010	2384/10014	150	1352/5677	1577/6623	2253/9463
154	1473/6185	1718/7216	2454/10308	154	1384/5814	1615/6783	2307/9690
158	1501/6302	1751/7353	2501/10504	158	1406/5905	1640/6889	2343/9842
162	1543/6479	1800/7559	2571/10798	162	1439/6042	1678/7049	2398/10070
166	1585/6655	1849/7764	2641/11092	166	1471/6179	1716/7209	2452/10298
170	1627/6832	1898/7970	2711/11386	170	1504/6316	1754/7368	2506/10526
174	1683/7067	1963/8245	2804/11778	174	1547/6498	1805/7581	2579/10830
178	1725/7243	2012/8450	2874/12072	178	1580/6635	1843/7741	2633/11058
182	1767/7420	2061/8656	2944/12366	182	1612/6772	1881/7900	2687/11286
186	1823/7655	2126/8913	3038/12758	186	1656/6954	1932/8113	2760/11590
190	1865/7831	2175/9136	3108/13052	190	1688/7091	1970/8273	2814/11818
194	1921/8066	2241/9411	3201/13444	194	1732/7273	2020/8485	2886/12122
198	1963/8243	2290/9617	3271/13738	198	1764/7410	2058/8645	2940/12350
202	2019/8478	2355/9891	3364/14130	202	1808/7592	2109/8858	3013/12654

	QUANTITY	CALS	KJ

BAKING

	QUANTITY	CALS	KJ
Almond Icing	25g	115	479
Almonds			
Flaked	10g	59	246
Ground	10g	59	246
Arrowroot	1 tsp	30	126
Baking Powder	1 tsp	10	42
Bicarbonate of Soda	1 tsp	0	0
Bran, Oat, *raw*	1 cup	231	967
Breadcrumbs	1 cup	250	1050
Chocolate Chips			
Cooking	100g	549	2305
Hail	28g	150	628
Cocoa Powder	1 tbsp	12	52
Coconut			
Desiccated	½ cup	12	52
Milk	200mL	437	1826
Condensed Milk, Sweetened	1 tbsp	70	293
Cornflour	1 tbsp	40	167
Cornmeal	100g	366	1530
Cream of Tartar	28g	72	302
Custard Powder	15g	91	381
Flour			
Gluten	100g	389	1622
Rice, White	100g	366	1530
Rye	100g	354	1480
Self-raising	100g	354	1480
Soya Bean	100g	436	1822
White	100g	351	1475
Wholemeal	100g	333	1394
Fruit Pectin	1 tbsp	3	13
Ghee (Clarified Butter)	1 tsp	44	184

BAKING

	QUANTITY	CALS	KJ
Ginger			
Crystallised	28g	95	399
Ground	1 tsp	6	26
Root, fresh	28g	22	94
Glucose Powder	1 tbsp	56	235
Golden Syrup	1 tsp	21	90
Hazelnuts	28g	176	735
Honey	1 tbsp	65	272
Icing Sugar	1 cup	467	1951
Lard	28g	252	1053
Lemon Juice, *fresh*	100mL	26	111
Lemon Peel	1 tsp	1	4
Lemon Rind, *grated*	28g	4	17
Lime Juice	1 tbsp	4	16
Maple Syrup	1 tbsp	52	518
Marzipan	28g	128	536
Minced Fruit	28g	47	198
Mustard Powder	1 tsp	15	65
Oatmeal	28g	112	469
Pastry			
Filo	per sheet	38	160
Puff	per sheet	452	1900
Shortcrust	28g	150	628
Peanuts, *raw*	1 cup	886	3720
Pearl Barley, *cooked*	1 cup	191	801
Pine Nuts	1 tbsp	60	252
Polenta	1 cup	505	2111
Poppy Seeds	10g	52	220
Semolina	28g	101	421
Shortening	1 tbsp	125	524
Spices, *ground*	1 tsp	5	21
Sugar			
Brown	1 cup	829	3467
White	1 cup	774	3235
Tahini	1 tbsp	101	424

	QUANTITY	CALS	KJ
Vinegar	1 tbsp	3	11
Walnuts, *shelled & chopped*	¼ cup	210	878
Wheatgerm	1 cup	414	1731
Yeast	1 tsp	12	49

BREAD

Bagels, Buns, Rolls & Muffins
ABE'S BAGEL BAKERY

Cinnamon Raisin	each	248	1040
Gluten Free	each	195	817
Mini	each	67	282
Multigrain	each	234	982
Natural	each	243	1020
Parmesan	each	250	1050
Sesame Seed	each	253	1060
GOLDEN			
Crumpet Breaks	each	118	494
Crumpets	each	95	398
English Muffins	each	145	607
Pikelets	each	109	457
HOMEBRAND			
Hamburger Buns	each	184	770
Hamburger Buns, Sesame	each	192	805
Long Rolls	each	184	770
Long Rolls, Sesame	each	206	865
NEW YORK BAGELS			
Blueberry	each	285	1196
Cin-Raisin	each	291	1220
Cranberry	each	296	1240
Mini	each	111	467
Onion	each	296	1240
Parmesan	each	293	1203
Plain	each	283	1185
Poppy	each	290	1215

BREAD

	QUANTITY	CALS	KJ
Sesame	each	291	1220
Wholemeal	each	297	1245
PAMS			
Burger Buns	each	191	800
King Buns	each	230	963
Long Rolls	each	192	805
Muffins			
Cheese	each	169	708
English	each	159	666
Spicy Fruit	each	175	734
Sesame Burger Buns	each	191	800
QUALITY BAKERS			
Crumpets	each	69	290
English Muffins			
Cheese	each	143	600
English	each	140	585
Spicy Fruit	each	139	580
Iced Finger Buns	each	45	190
Nature's Fresh			
Burger Buns	each	186	780
Burger Buns, Sesame	each	193	810
Hot Dog Rolls	each	186	780
King Burger Buns	each	234	980
Long Rolls	each	186	780
Long Rolls, Wholemeal	each	176	740
Pikelets	each	65	270
SIGNATURE RANGE			
Bagels			
Original	each	241	1010
Sesame	each	255	1070
English Muffins			
Cheese	each	143	597
English	each	102	425
Spicy Fruit	each	139	580

	QUANTITY	CALS	KJ
TIP TOP			
Muffins			
Cheese	each	169	708
English	each	158	662
Spicy Fruit	each	176	734
Oatilicious, Long Rolls	each	195	865
Super Soft			
Plain White Burger Buns	each	192	803
Plain White Long Rolls	each	192	803
Sesame Burger Buns	each	192	803
Sesame Long Rolls	each	192	803
Sliced White King Buns	each	230	963
VENERDI			
Toasting Baps	per slice	163	685
WAFFLE ONS			
Choc Chip	each	211	879
Vanilla	each	235	985
Sliced			
BAKEWORKS			
Liberté			
Grain Sustain	per slice	96	403
Original	per slice	95	398
Sunflower & Linseed	per slice	102	427
Wholemeal	per slice	98	411
White Farmhouse Loaf	per slice	70	293
BÜRGEN			
Fruit Toast	per slice	95	400
Grains with Barley Toast	per slice	102	427
Mixed Grain Sandwich	per slice	78	327
Mixed Grain Toast	per slice	87	367
Pumpkin Seed & Chia Toast	per slice	103	432
Soy & Linseed Sandwich	per slice	94	384
Soy & Linseed Toast	per slice	92	384
Wholemeal & Seeds Toast	per slice	108	450

BREAD

	QUANTITY	CALS	KJ
FREYA'S			
Dutch Wholemeal Grain	per slice	99	415
Quinoa & Flaxseed	per slice	104	435
Roggenbrot Dark Rye	per slice	100	420
Sunflower & Barley	per slice	110	460
Swiss Soya Linseed	per slice	112	470
Tuscan Mixed Grain	per slice	107	450
HOMEBRAND			
White Bread	per slice	78	327
Wholemeal Toast	per slice	67	310
MACKENZIE HIGH COUNTRY BREAD			
Original White	per slice	164	690
Southern Grain	per slice	148	620
Station Seed & Grain	per slice	155	650
Stone Ground Wholemeal	per slice	148	620
Tussock Hills Malted Grain	per slice	150	630
MOLENBERG			
Balance			
Sandwich	per slice	68	285
Toast	per slice	82	345
Grains Plus Toast	per slice	89	375
Hidden Grains	per slice	81	340
Original			
Sandwich	per slice	70	295
Toast	per slice	86	360
Vitality			
Sandwich	per slice	75	315
Toast	per slice	92	385
PAMS			
Delicious Traditional Mixed Grain	per slice	91	384
Multigrain Sandwich	per slice	74	311
Multigrain Toast	per slice	90	378
Wheatmeal Sandwich	per slice	75	314
Wheatmeal Toast	per slice	91	381
White Sandwich	per slice	76	319

	QUANTITY	CALS	KJ
White Toast	per slice	92	387
Wholesome Traditional Soy & Linseed	per slice	95	398
Scrumptious Traditional White	per slice	88	369
PAVILLION			
Chia Seed	per slice	121	510
Gluten Free Original	per slice	119	500
Original	per slice	120	505
Soy & Linseed	per slice	118	494
PLOUGHMANS BAKERY			
Country Grains	per slice	106	445
Farmhouse Wholemeal	per slice	103	432
Harvest Light Rye	per slice	106	445
Rustic White	per slice	106	445
Soy & Canterbury Linseed	per slice	111	466
Wholemeal & Grains	per slice	100	417
SIGNATURE RANGE			
Highland Rye Toast	per slice	84	355
Highland Wholemeal Toast	per slice	85	357
Mixed Grain Toast	per slice	110	463
Multigrain Sandwich	per slice	66	280
Multigrain Toast	per slice	83	340
Soy & Linseed Toast	per slice	96	405
Wheatmeal Sandwich	per slice	69	290
Wheatmeal Toast	per slice	84	352
White Sandwich	per slice	59	250
White Toast	per slice	71	301
TIP TOP			
Goodness Grains			
9 Grain & Seed Toast	per slice	96	403
Original Swiss Sandwich	per slice	71	299
Original Swiss Toast	per slice	86	362
Soy & Linseed Toast	per slice	94	396
Sunflower & Chia Toast	per slice	94	396
Oatilicious, Toast	per slice	93	388
Super Soft			

BREAD

	QUANTITY	CALS	KJ
Honey Grain Toast	per slice	91	381
Multigrain Toast	per slice	90	377
White Sandwich	per slice	76	320
White Super Thick	per slice	118	493
White Toast	per slice	93	388
Wholemeal Sandwich	per slice	73	304
Wholemeal Toast	per slice	88	369
The One			
Sandwich	per slice	71	297
Toast	per slice	86	360
TWO HANDS			
Great White Sourdough	per slice	73	477
Mixed Grain with Pumpkin Seeds	per slice	118	496
VENERDI			
Gluten Free Range			
Ancient Multi Grain	per slice	102	430
Full Flavour Six Seeds	per slice	106	444
Original Brown Rice	per slice	100	420
VOGEL'S			
Gluten Free			
6 Seed	per slice	101	425
Chia & Toasted Sesame	per slice	82	345
Fruit & Spice	per slice	95	400
Soy & Linseed	per slice	96	405
Sunflower & Red Quinoa	per slice	88	370
White	per slice	81	340
Original			
Ancient Grains Toast	per slice	99	415
Chia & Toasted Sesame Toast	per slice	93	392
Original Mixed Grain Sandwich	per slice	77	325
Original Mixed Grain Toast	per slice	95	400
Original Mixed Grain Very Thin Cut	per slice	63	265
Soft Mixed Grain Sandwich	per slice	77	325
Soy & Linseed Toast	per slice	103	435
Spelt & Flaxseed Toast	per slice	97	410

	QUANTITY	CALS	KJ
Sunflower & Barley Toast	per slice	108	455
Speciality Bread			
BAZAAR			
Chilled Garlic & Cheese Loaf	per slice	144	604
Chilled Garlic Double Baguette	per slice	137	577
Chilled Garlic Loaf	51g	174	730
Chilled Garlic Single Baguette	25g	76	318
Garlic Bread	per slice	67	282
Gourmet Pizza Bases	110g	319	1338
Traditional Roti	each	128	536
White Tortilla	each	192	804
Wholemeal Tortilla	each	194	810
DANNY'S			
Fresh Daily Pita Bread			
Garlic Filled	each	246	1035
Garlic Filled Wholemeal	each	246	1035
Lebanese	each	105	440
Olive Filled	each	244	1027
Original	each	105	440
Wholemeal	each	105	440
Long Life Pita Bread			
Garlic Filled	each	246	1035
Garlic Filled Wholemeal	each	246	1035
Oat Bran Mini	each	108	452
Olive Filled	each	244	1027
Original	each	105	440
Original Mini	each	105	440
Wholemeal	each	105	440
Wholemeal Mini	each	105	440
Mediterranean Bread			
Basil, Oregano & Paprika Italian Bread	each	124	520
Cardamom & Fennel Turkish Bread	each	124	520
Cumin & Coriander Moroccan Bread	each	124	520

BREAD

	QUANTITY	CALS	KJ
DISCOVERY			
Tortillas			
Chilli & Jalapenos	each	131	552
Corn	each	119	500
Garlic & Herb	each	117	494
Large Flour	each	153	646
Plain Flour	each	118	497
Preservative Free	each	130	549
Wholemeal	each	109	460
FARRAH WRAPS			
Fire Roasted Pepper	each	224	938
Garden Spinach	each	225	945
Multigrain	each	225	945
Premium White	each	224	938
Wellness High Fibre White	each	155	650
Wellness Sunflower & Linseed	each	149	625
Wholemeal	each	223	937
FREYA'S			
Pitas			
Garlic & Herb	each	371	1550
Soy & Linseed	each	285	1190
Wraps			
Oats & Barley Round	each	157	660
Original	each	174	730
Soy Linseed Round	each	148	620
OLD EL PASO			
Healthy Fiesta, Extra Light Tortilla	each	120	503
Mini Tortilla	each	86	360
Tortilla	each	135	568
PAMS			
Naan, Garlic Flat Breads, Indian Style	each	168	703
Naan, Plain Flat Breads, Indian Style	each	165	694
Panini, Plain Breads, Italian Style	each	274	1150
Pita Bread			
Garlic	each	110	464

	QUANTITY	CALS	KJ
White	each	107	449
Wholemeal	each	112	471
Wrap, Spinach Flat Breads, Mediterranean Style	each	139	585
Wrap, White Flat Breads, Mediterranean Style	each	135	567
PAVILLION			
Pizza Base	each	528	2210
Tortillas	each	209	878
POSEY, Original	50g	126	529
SIGNATURE RANGE, Pita	50g	130	540
TURKISH BREAD			
Garlic Bread	73g	202	847
Garlic Bread, Gourmet Cheesy	71g	203	850
Garlic Bread, Twin Pack	73g	214	897
Thin & Crispy, Pre-Sauced Pizza Base	112g	192	807
Turkish Naan, Buttered Garlic	100g	276	1160
Wood-Fired Pizza Bases, Thin & Crispy	75g	197	825
WATTLE VALLEY			
Lite White	each	110	461
Sourdough	each	126	527
Wheat & Rye	each	129	538
Wholegrain	each	117	490

Breakfast Cereal, Porridge & Muesli

ALISON'S PANTRY

Almond & Orange Berry Clusters	50g	250	1046
Ancient Grains & Cinnamon Clusters	50g	225	943
Best Breakfast	50g	161	675
Black Forest Clusters	50g	245	1026
Bran	50g	133	560
Bran & Sultana Cereal	50g	166	693
Bulgur Wheat	50g	176	739
Cornflakes	50g	182	765

BREAKFAST CEREAL, PORRIDGE & MUESLI

	QUANTITY	CALS	KJ
Cranberry Crunch Muesli	50g	179	753
Date & Hazelnut Bircher Muesli	50g	197	825
Instant Oats	50g	160	670
Lecithin	50g	387	1622
Multi Bran	50g	148	620
Natural Muesli	50g	181	760
Oatbran	50g	160	670
Raw Power	50g	232	974
Swiss Toasted Muesli	50g	199	833
Toasted Muesli	50g	176	737
Wheatgerm	50g	161	675
Whole Grain Oats	50g	160	670
Yoghurt & Berry Crunch	50g	192	807
BE NATURAL			
5 Whole Grain Flakes	45g	164	690
Cashew, Almond, Hazelnut & Coconut	45g	193	810
Manuka Honey & Spice Clusters	45g	172	720
Pink Lady Apple & Flame Raisin	45g	169	710
BROOKFARM			
Macadamia Muesli			
Gluten Free	35g	155	651
Natural with Apricots & Apples	50g	205	863
Natural with Cranberries	50g	207	866
Toasted with Apricots	50g	222	932
Toasted with Cranberries	50g	221	925
BUDGET			
Cocoa Puffs	30g	116	489
Cornflakes	30g	111	465
Tropical Muesli	50g	167	700
CARMAN'S			
Classic Fruit & Nut Muesli	45g	203	851
Original Fruit Free Muesli	45g	217	909
CERES ORGANICS			
Amaranth, Puffed	35g	130	544

BREAKFAST CEREAL, PORRIDGE & MUESLI

	QUANTITY	CALS	KJ
Cereal			
Buckwheat	50g	171	718
Millet	60g	226	949
Quinoa	40g	163	686
Rice	60g	207	869
Muesli			
Apricot & Almond	50g	215	901
Bircher Original	50g	190	798
Gluten Free	50g	210	879
Golden Crunch	50g	227	905
Honey Toasted	50g	206	866
Tropical	50g	202	849
Oats			
Jumbo Rolled Oats Wholegrain	50g	192	804
Oat Bran	50g	123	515
Rolled Oats	50g	192	804
Quinoa Flakes	42g	172	720
Quinoa Puffs	35g	128	539
FREEDOM FOODS			
Ancient Grain Flakes	50g	187	783
Ancient Grain Super Muesli	50g	207	870
Corn Flakes	50g	198	829
Ultra Rice Maple Crunch	45g	170	712
GOODNESS SUPERFOODS			
Digestive	50g	163	690
Heart First	50g	144	815
GRAIN HEALTH PRODUCTS			
Almond Crumble Muesli	50g	221	925
Original Muesli	50g	224	935
Sunrise Caramel	30g	116	487
Sweet Maple	40g	116	487
GRAIN PRODUCTS, Vita-Brits	30g	106	444
HARRAWAYS			
Fruit Harvest	45g	149	608

BREAKFAST CEREAL, PORRIDGE & MUESLI

	QUANTITY	CALS	KJ
Oat Singles			
Apple, Sultana & Cinnamon	40g	134	564
Honey & Golden Syrup	30g	102	427
Original	40g	128	536
Organic Rolled Oats	40g	152	640
Organic Wholegrain Oats	40g	129	536
Rolled Oats	45g	144	603
Scotch Oats	45g	144	603
Traditional Wholegrain	40g	129	536
HEALTHERIES			
Bircher Muesli			
Apple & Raisin	74g	294	1230
Apple & Raspberry Flakes	71g	276	1160
Deluxe	70g	276	1150
Simple			
Apricot & Raisin Wholegrain Hot Cereal	50g	174	729
Berry Light Cereal	45g	170	710
Hi-Fibre Muesli	66g	257	1080
Honey Flakes	45g	167	703
Tropical Light Cereal	51g	189	791
HILLARY FOODS			
Cereal & Nuggets	40g	149	624
Cereal & Nuggets, Banana Honey	40g	151	632
HOMEBRAND			
Bran & Sultanas	45g	153	644
Cocoa Puffs	30g	116	489
Corn Flakes	30g	108	456
Fruit & Nut Muesli	50g	198	830
Honey Poppas	30g	118	496
Oatbran	20g	76	320
Quick Oats	30g	114	477
Rice Pops	30g	113	474
Rolled Oats	30g	114	477
Traditional Muesli	50g	190	790
Wheat Biscuits	30g	105	441

	QUANTITY	CALS	KJ
HUBBARDS			
Bran			
Bran & Berries	45g	163	680
Bran & Clusters	45g	177	740
Bran & Sultana	45g	164	684
Brantastix	45g	145	605
Kids			
Banana Bugs'n'Mud	30g	176	445
Berry Tricks Mix	30g	117	490
Cookies & Cream Rumbles	30g	119	500
Cornflakes	30g	112	465
Neapolitan Super Pops	30g	115	483
Light & Right			
Apricot	45g	174	729
Berry	45g	171	716
Feijoa	45g	167	702
Hazelnut & Almond	45g	179	752
Passionfruit	45g	171	716
Muesli			
Original			
Berry Berry Lite	45g	171	716
Berry Berry Nice	50g	199	835
Clever Clusters	45g	189	792
Fruitful Breakfast	50g	201	845
Fruitful Lite	45g	173	725
The Amazing Range			
Double Toasted Golden Syrup & Cranberry	50g	195	819
Lightly Toasted Apricot & Papaya	50g	182	765
Natural 5 Fruits & Honey	50g	176	740
Natural 5 Grains & Hazelnut	50g	193	810
Toasted Almond & Pecan	50g	217	910
Toasted Pomegranate & Blueberry	50g	204	855
Simply			
Clusters Berry	50g	215	900

BREAKFAST CEREAL, PORRIDGE & MUESLI

	QUANTITY	CALS	KJ
Natural Berry	50g	188	790
Natural Fruit & Nut	50g	201	845
Reduced Fat Cranberry & Vanilla	50g	198	830
Toasted Apricot	50g	201	840
Toasted Nuts & Seeds	50g	205	860
Toasted Original	50g	212	885
Outward Bound	45g	167	702
Thank Goodness Gluten Free			
Apricot & Apple Muesli	45g	172	720
Berry Muesli	45g	169	710
Brown Rice Porridge, Cinnamon	35g	133	560
Brown Rice Porridge, Maple	35g	131	550
Cocoa Puffs	30g	120	501
Cornflakes	30g	114	477
Original	30g	114	480
Rice Pops	30g	115	485
Vanilla Almond Muesli	45g	184	770
KELLOGG'S			
All-Bran			
Apple Flavoured Crunch	45g	162	680
Original	45g	148	620
Wheat Flakes Honey Almond	45g	164	690
Wheat Flakes Original	40g	136	570
Coco Pops	30g	114	480
Coco Pops Chex	30g	112	470
Corn Flakes	30g	112	470
Crispix	30g	117	490
Crunchy Nut			
Clusters	30g	124	520
Corn Flakes	30g	119	500
Froot Loops	30g	117	490
Frosties	30g	114	480
Guardian	30g	102	430
Just Right			
Antioxidant	45g	162	680

	QUANTITY	CALS	KJ
Clusters & 5 Grains	45g	160	670
Original	45g	169	710
Mini-Wheats			
5 Grains	40g	143	600
Blackcurrant	40g	143	600
Mixed Berry Flavour	40g	138	580
Nutri-Grain	30g	114	480
Rice Bubbles	30g	114	480
Special K			
Advantage	40g	141	590
Forest Berries	30g	112	470
Fruit & Nut Medley	40g	155	650
Honey Almond	30g	119	500
Original	30g	112	470
Sultana Bran			
Original	45g	152	640
Sultana Bran Buds	45g	150	630
Sultana Bran Extra	45g	157	660
Sustain	45g	169	710
LOWAN			
Cocoa Bombs	35g	140	570
Muesli			
Apple & Cinnamon	45g	173	720
Apricot & Almond	45g	172	729
Fruit & Nut	45g	171	707
Light	45g	166	693
Original Harvest	45g	180	756
Swiss	45g	163	708
Tropical Fruit	45g	175	729
Oats			
Natural Oat Bran	40g	149	625
Quick Oats	30g	115	483
Rolled Oats	30g	115	483
Rice Flakes	55g	199	831
Rice Porridge	50g	178	743

BREAKFAST CEREAL, PORRIDGE & MUESLI

	QUANTITY	CALS	KJ
NATURE'S PATH ORGANIC			
Corn Flakes Fruit Juice Sweetened	30g	120	504
Crispy Rice Cereal	30g	110	460
Heritage Flakes	30g	120	502
Honey'd Corn Flakes	30g	120	502
Mesa Sunrise Flakes	30g	120	502
Millet Rice Flakes	30g	120	502
Multigrain Oatbran Flakes	30g	110	460
Oaty Bites	30g	110	460
Optimum Blueberry Cinnamon Flax Cereal	55g	200	836
Smartbran Cereal	30g	80	334
Spelt Flakes	30g	110	460
Sunrise Crunchy Maple	30g	110	460
NESTLÉ			
MILO Cereal	30g	116	493
MILO Crunchy Bites	30g	114	480
MILO Duo Cereal	30g	117	490
NESQUIK Cereal	30g	114	480
NICOLA'S ORGANIC MUESLI			
96% Fat Free Toasted	30g	91	383
Gluten Free Wheat Free Toasted	30g	118	496
Manuka Honey Toasted	30g	97	410
Oat Singles Plain	30g	152	640
Unsweetened	30g	111	466
PAMS			
Bran & Sultana	30g	101	426
Corn Flakes	30g	111	465
Creamy Porridge	45g	144	603
Fruity Loops	30g	108	455
Honey Snaps	30g	119	498
Instant Oat Sachets			
Brown Sugar & Honey	35g	135	567
Cranberry & Apple	35g	134	564

	QUANTITY	CALS	KJ
Lite & Fruity			
Apricot Fruit	45g	156	653
Mixed Berry	45g	158	662
Tropical Mix	45g	157	657
Muesli			
Natural	50g	198	830
Toasted	50g	204	855
Rice Snaps	30g	114	477
Rolled Oats	45g	144	603
Wheat Biskits	2 biscuits	105	441
Wholegrain Oats	40g	127	536
PUREBREAD			
Inca Gold Crunchies	40g	156	656
Wild Oats Muesli	75g	314	1320
SANITARIUM			
Cluster Crisp			
Caramel Latte	50g	213	890
Honey with Roasted Cashew	50g	219	915
Triple Berry	50g	210	865
Vanilla Almond	50g	218	910
Grains To Go			
Apricot	35g	146	609
Berry	35g	143	599
Original	35g	147	616
Fibre Life Bran Flakes	45g	125	522
Honey Puffs	30g	115	480
Light 'n' Tasty			
Apricot	45g	166	693
Berry Fruits	45g	156	655
Macadamia	45g	188	752
Manuka Honey, Date & Nut	45g	170	710
Peach & Raspberry	45g	166	695
Plum & Almond	45g	168	700
Muesli			
Lite Muesli Plum & Cranberry	45g	173	725

BREAKFAST CEREAL, PORRIDGE & MUESLI

	QUANTITY	CALS	KJ
Natural Muesli Fruit & 5 Grains	50g	188	785
Toasted Muesli Cranberry & Almond	50g	209	875
Toasted Muesli Golden Oats & Fruit	50g	214	895
Toasted Muesli Hi Fibre	45g	187	785
Toasted Muesli Nuts & Seeds	50g	227	950
Toasted Muesli Strawberry & Rhubarb	50g	209	875
Toasted Muesli Super Fruity	50g	204	850
Puffed Wheat	25g	93	390
Ricies	30g	114	477
San Bran	45g	134	558
Skippy Cornflakes	30g	111	465
Weet-Bix			
Energize	50g	187	780
Hi-Bran	40g	143	596
Multi-Grain	48g	184	768
Oat Bran	40g	144	604
Original	30g	105	441
Weet-Bix Bites			
Apricot	45g	154	644
Berry	45g	157	657
Crunch Honey	45g	169	707
Energize	45g	169	707
Rough Crumble	45g	179	747
Weeties	30g	108	450
SELECT			
Clusters			
Berry	45g	167	702
Vanilla Almond	45g	175	729
Great Start	45g	167	702
Great Start, Berry	45g	167	702
Morning Crunch Muesli	50g	219	915
SIGNATURE RANGE			
Wheat Biscuits	30g	105	441
UNCLE TOBYS			
Cheerios	30g	117	490

	QUANTITY	CALS	KJ
Honey Cheerios	30g	117	490
Milk Oaties	40g	151	870
Oat Crisps			
Almond	40g	162	680
Hazelnut	40g	162	680
Oats Quick Sachets			
Brown Sugar & Cinnamon	35g	133	560
Creamy Honey	35g	136	570
Creamy Vanilla	35g	133	560
Golden Syrup	35g	133	560
Original	35g	129	540
VOGEL'S			
All Good			
Almond, Cashew & Linseed	50g	201	845
Apple Crunch	50g	192	805
Golden Crunch	50g	201	845
Café-Style			
Light Almond & Ancient Grains	45g	191	801
Light Berry	40g	150	669
Light Crisp Clusters with Cranberries	45g	157	660
Light Luxury Nuts & Seeds	45g	187	783
Light Vanilla & Almond	40g	170	712
Luxury Muesli	47g	198	830
Porridge, Banana & Pecan	45g	175	735
Cranberry & Blackcurrant Clusters	45g	177	743
Crunchy Honey Clusters	45g	179	752
Luxury Blend			
Cranberry, Cashew & Pistachio	50g	220	921
Macadamia, Date & Honey	50g	205	861
Maple, Walnut & Almond	50g	230	966
WEIGHT WATCHERS			
Berry Flakes	45g	158	662
Fruit & Fibre Tropical	45g	162	680
Fruity Muesli	45g	174	729
Oven Baked Berry Muesli	45g	166	698

	QUANTITY	CALS	KJ
Oven Baked Nutty Muesli	45g	171	716

Cakes & Slices

	QUANTITY	CALS	KJ
AUNT BETTY'S, Raspberry Tarts	33g	155	651
BALCONI			
Mix Max	each	150	627
Rollino			
Cocoa	each	160	669
Milk	each	160	669
Tiramisu	100g	364	1522
CAKEMARK			
Cake Bars, *The Simpsons*	28g	96	406
Chocolate Mini Rolls	each	114	477
Chow Bars, *The Simpsons*	30g	138	579
Coconut Delights	42g	193	808
Large Coconut Macaroons	100g	417	1746
DELMAINE			
Almond Delights	47g	175	735
Almond Fingers	43g	172	720
Almond Rounds	47g	193	809
Apple Rounds	47g	180	755
Coconut Stars	12g	52	221
ERNEST ADAMS			
Cakes			
Apricot & Sultana Loaf	40g	124	520
Banana & Choc Chip Loaf	40g	150	630
Date & Walnut Loaf	40g	124	520
Fruit Cake	40g	143	600
Jamaican Ginger Loaf	40g	143	600
Madeira Cake	35g	136	570
Sultana Cake	45g	167	700
Un-filled Sponge	38g	131	550
Gluten Free			
Caramel	44g	205	860

	QUANTITY	CALS	KJ
Chocolate Brownie	44g	210	880
Chocolate Cake	44g	186	780
Jamaican Ginger Cake	41g	157	660
Lemon Cake	44g	181	760
Raspberry Slice	44g	193	810
Slices			
Apricot	38g	141	590
Caramel	38g	179	750
Fruit	38g	152	640
Ginger	38g	193	810
Louise	38g	160	670
Raspberry	38g	164	690
Russian	38g	184	770
PAVILLION			
Belgium Slice	55g	228	957
Fudge Slice	55g	226	947
ROSEDALE			
Ginger Kisses	each	102	429
Lemon Kisses	each	102	429
Maple Walnut Kisses	each	107	446
SIGNATURE RANGE			
Chocolate Kisses	each	102	425
Ginger Kisses	each	103	430
WEIGHT WATCHERS			
Carrot Cake Slice	22g	68	285
Chocolate Mini Rolls	23g	90	378

Chocolate Products

ALISON'S PANTRY			
Caramel Bites	50g	218	913
Choc Hokey Pokey	50g	215	900
Choc Minnows	50g	187	785
Chocolate Caramel	50g	250	1050
Chocolate Chunks	25g	124	519

CHOCOLATE PRODUCTS

	QUANTITY	CALS	KJ
Chocolate Fudge	50g	212	891
Chocolate Pineapple Pieces	50g	218	915
Chocolate Pretzels	50g	241	1011
Coconut Rough	50g	262	1098
Dark Chocolate Ginger	50g	201	843
Hokey Pokey Clusters (Chocolate)	50g	265	1112
Milk Chocolate Almonds	50g	271	1135
Milk Chocolate Peanuts	50g	273	1145
Milk Chocolate Raisins	50g	229	960
Peanut Minis (Chocolate)	50g	286	1198
Roses Chocolates	100g	480	2010
Strawberry Dream (Chocolate)	50g	272	1140
Tri Chocolate Strawberries	30g	146	614
CADBURY			
Bars			
Buzz	per bar	82	346
Chocolate Fish	per bar	78	330
Crunchie	per bar	241	1010
Curly Wurly	per bar	116	489
Flake	per bar	162	681
Freddo	10g	53	334
Fry's Turkish Delight	15g	54	228
Moro	100g	207	870
Moro Gold	60g	306	1284
Moro Gold Stix	per bar	299	1284
Picnic	per bar	241	1010
Pinky	per bar	152	639
Blocks			
Black Forest	25g	127	533
Caramello	25g	122	514
Coconut Rough	25g	138	581
Crunchie	25g	122	512
Dairy Milk	25g	133	559
Dream	25g	140	587
Duo	per piece	32	136

	QUANTITY	CALS	KJ
Energy	25g	131	549
Fruit & Nut	25g	126	531
Hazelnut	25g	139	584
Old Gold 70% Cocoa	25g	136	571
Old Gold Jamaica Rum 'n' Raisin	25g	122	513
Old Gold Original	25g	130	546
Old Gold Peppermint	25g	113	175
Old Gold Roast Almond	25g	134	564
Rocky Road	25g	133	557
Snack	25g	116	489
Top Deck	25g	136	570
Turkish Delight	25g	113	473
Boxes			
Favourites	25g	121	509
Milk Tray	25g	122	512
Old Gold	25g	115	485
Roses	25g	114	481
Marvellous Creations			
Banana Candy Peanut Drops Choc Biscuit	25g	128	536
Jelly Crunchie Bits	25g	122	513
Jelly Popping Candy Beanies	25g	127	534
Peanut Toffee Cookie	25g	123	518
Toblerone	25g	132	454
FERRERO ROCHER	each	74	310
GREEN & BLACK'S ORGANIC			
Dark 85%	25g	160	655
Maya Gold	25g	140	570
Milk Chocolate	25g	140	560
GUYLIAN			
Blocks			
Dark 72%	100g	516	2159
Dark No Sugar	100g	465	1946
Milk	100g	498	2082
Milk & Almond	100g	554	2320

CHOCOLATE PRODUCTS

	QUANTITY	CALS	KJ
Milk & Hazelnut	100g	564	2360
La Trufflina	each	68	288
Opus	each	74	311
Sea Shell	each	62	260
HERSHEY'S			
Bars			
Cookies 'n' Creme	per bar	220	920
Milk Chocolate	per bar	210	878
Milk Chocolate with Almonds	per bar	210	878
Special Dark	per bar	190	795
Chocolate Kisses			
Creamy Milk Chocolate	each	24	103
Dark Chocolate	each	21	90
Milk Chocolate filled with Caramel	each	22	90
Milk Chocolate with Almonds	each	23	97
KINDER SURPRISE	each	230	469
LINDT			
Creations			
Divine Hazelnut	20g	109	457
Heavenly Crème Brulée	20g	115	484
Sumptuous Orange	20g	106	444
Velvety Vanilla Almond	20g	112	471
Excellence			
70% Cocoa	40g	208	872
85% Cocoa	40g	228	954
Blueberry Intense	40g	200	840
Chili Chocolate	40g	202	848
Coconut Intense	25g	127	532
Creamy Milk Hazelnut	25g	142	595
Extra Creamy	40g	223	936
Milk	40g	224	936
Mint Intense	40g	218	460
Orange Intense	40g	216	908
Passionfruit Intense	25g	126	530
White	25g	141	593

	QUANTITY	CALS	KJ
Lindor			
Caramel	22g	138	580
Extra Dark	22g	138	580
Milk	2 pieces	154	645
MALTESERS	25g	125	525
MARS			
Bounty Bar	100g	482	2020
M&Ms			
Crispy	25g	122	513
Milk Chocolate	25g	122	513
Peanut	25g	127	535
Raspberry	25g	121	510
Mars Bar	each	243	1020
Milky Way	each	444	1860
Snickers	each	260	1090
Twix	each	504	2110
NESTLÉ			
Bars			
Aero, Caramel	20g	102	429
Aero, Chocolate	20g	108	451
Aero, Mint	20g	107	450
Bounty	per bar	108	456
Chokito	per bar	259	1085
Kit Kat	2 fingers	117	490
Kit Kat Chunky	2 fingers	105	440
Kit Kat Chunky, Caramel	2 fingers	114	480
Kit Kat Chunky, Cookies & Cream	100g	121	490
Pixie Caramel	50g	231	970
King-Size Blocks			
Kit Kat	100g	523	2190
Kit Kat White	15g	83	350
Milky Bar	25g	139	583
Milky Bar, Milk & Cookies	22g	121	510
Rolo	20g	100	420
Smarties	100g	525	2200

CHOCOLATE PRODUCTS

	QUANTITY	CALS	KJ
Scorched Almonds	24g	121	510
Scorched Almonds, White	24g	126	530
Smarties	100g	478	2000
Wonka Blocks			
Caramel Hat Trick	100g	509	2130
Nutty Crunchilicious	100g	537	2250
Triple Chocolate Wipple	100g	523	2190
RICHFIELDS			
Classic Dark	20g	118	495
Superfine Milk	20g	114	480
SENZ			
Dark Chocolate	20g	114	476
Milk Chocolate	20g	111	464
Milk Chocolate Caramel	20g	109	454
WELL NATURALLY			
Sugar Free Mint Crisp	15g	68	284
Sugar Free Rich Dark	15g	71	297
WHITTAKER'S			
Blocks			
Almond Gold	25g	143	601
Berry & Biscuit	25g	125	523
Coconut	25g	145	607
Creamy Milk	25g	140	589
Dark	25g	136	571
Dark Almond	25g	137	574
Dark Cacao	25g	132	553
Dark Caramel	25g	117	491
Dark Ghana	25g	138	580
Dark Orange	25g	129	541
Fruit & Nut	25g	134	562
Ghana Peppermint	25g	122	514
Hazelnut	25g	146	615
Hokey Pokey	25g	130	545
Kiwifruit	25g	127	535
L&P	25g	133	559

	QUANTITY	CALS	KJ
Macadamia	25g	146	612
Milk Caramel	25g	122	514
Milk Madagascar	25g	133	558
Milk Strawberry	25g	120	503
Peanut	25g	139	586
Peanut Butter	25g	142	595
Rum & Raisin	25g	121	509
White Chocolate	25g	135	568
White Macadamia	25g	141	594
White Raspberry	25g	135	565
Chunks Bars			
Cashew Nut	50g	284	1190
Creamy Milk	50g	281	1177
Dark Chunks	50g	272	1142
Dark Ghana	50g	277	1160
Dark Orange	50g	258	1080
Fruit & Nut	50g	268	1125
White Chocolate	50g	279	1170
Mini Slab			
Almond & Cranberry	each	78	327
Almond Gold	each	86	361
Berry & Biscuit	each	75	314
Coconut	each	87	365
Cornflake	each	80	335
Creamy Milk	each	84	353
Dark Peppermint	each	81	343
Hokey Pokey	each	79	333
L&P	each	80	336
Peanut	each	79	333
White Raspberry	each	81	339
Slabs			
Almond Gold	50g	263	1103
Berry & Biscuit	50g	249	1045
Coconut	50g	298	1248
Creamy Milk	50g	281	1177

CHOCOLATE PRODUCTS/CONFECTIONERY

	QUANTITY	CALS	KJ
Dark Peanut	50g	279	1170
Hazelnut	50g	237	995
Hokey Pokey	50g	260	1090
L&P	50g	267	1120
Peanut	50g	282	1184
Raisin & Peanut	50g	260	1091
Super Almond Gold 70g	70g	401	1680
Super Dark Peanut 75g	75g	418	1750
Super Peanut 75g	75g	282	1184
Squares			
Creamy Milk	each	59	247
Dark	each	58	242
Dark Ghana	each	59	248
Dark Peppermint	each	57	240

Confectionery

ALISON'S PANTRY

Black Balls	50g	192	805
Butterflies	50g	167	700
Caribbean Treat	50g	170	715
Carob Mushrooms	20g	91	383
Coconut Ice	50g	95	401
Cranberry Nut Nougat	25g	105	442
Crocodiles	50g	161	674
English Style Winegums	50g	168	706
Fairy Mushrooms	40g	165	692
Fruit Rascals	50g	185	775
Giant Pythons	50g	155	650
Giant Strawberries	50g	176	738
Gum Balls	50g	193	810
Gummi Bears	50g	178	745
Gummi Pirates	50g	190	795
Jellybeans	50g	193	808
Jersey Caramels	50g	200	840

	QUANTITY	CALS	KJ
Jumbo Jellybeans	50g	193	808
Jumbo Marshmallows	35g	121	508
Kool Bananas	50g	166	697
Licorice Allsorts	50g	186	780
Lolly Scramble	50g	209	875
Love Hearts	50g	172	720
Mega Allsorts	50g	186	780
Milk Bottles	50g	184	770
Mini Fruits	50g	187	785
Party Mix	50g	171	719
Planes	50g	168	705
Rainbow Buttons	50g	239	1000
Raspberries & Blackberries	50g	159	667
Russian Fudge	50g	210	880
Sherbet Fizzies	50g	187	783
Soft Jubes	50g	174	732
Sour Hearts	50g	167	700
Sour Jaw Breakers	50g	190	796
Sour Lollies	50g	170	712
Sour Rainbow Belts	25g	86	360
Strawberry & Cream	50g	168	705
Super Ojays	50g	244	1025
Supreme Nougat	25g	110	462
Tangy Apple Pipes	25g	88	372
Tangy Sticks	50g	190	798
Yoghurt Fruities	50g	165	694
Yum Skulls	50g	164	690
ALLEN'S			
Allsorts	10g	36	154
Jellies			
Jelly Beans	20g	76	320
Party Mix	20g	69	290
Snakes Alive	20g	66	280
Kool Fruits	20g	77	326
Lollipops	each	31	130

CONFECTIONERY

	QUANTITY	CALS	KJ
Mackintosh's Toffees	15g	62	262
Mints			
Kool Mints	20g	75	315
Kool Mints, Spearmint	20g	74	314
Oddfellows Chewy	20g	74	310
Oddfellows Mint	20g	40	170
Oddfellows Smokers	20g	81	340
Oddfellows Spearmint	20g	81	340
Redskins	each	47	200
BEACON, Liquorice Allsorts	25g	94	396
BLACK KNIGHT, Liquorice	30g	105	440
CADBURY			
Caramels	25g	123	518
Fudge Duets	25g	109	460
Jaffas	25g	122	513
Pebbles	25g	115	484
CHUPA CHUPS, The Best Of	each	147	195
DOUBLE 'D'			
Butter	each	8	36
Fruit	each	7	32
Lemon 'n' Lime	each	7	32
HARIBO			
Gold Bears	40g	139	584
Happy Cola	40g	139	584
Starmix	40g	139	584
Tangfastics	40g	138	580
HEARDS			
Barley Sugar	each	17	75
Fruit Refreshers	each	17	74
HOMEBRAND			
Airplanes	20g	72	302
Black Jelly Beans	20g	76	320
Crown Mints	6g	24	101
Jelly Beans	20g	76	320
Jersey Caramels	20g	82	344

	QUANTITY	CALS	KJ
Kiwi Party Mix	20g	76	320
Marshmallows	25g	88	372
Pineapple Pieces	20g	86	364
Sour Worms	10g	36	153
JELLY BELLY			
Assorted	40g	148	620
Sours	40g	145	608
Sunkist	40g	145	608
KIWILANDS, Barley Sugars	15g	58	246
MACEYS, Lollipops	each	13	56
MENTOS			
Mint	10g	139	165
New Rainbow	10g	39	64
MR MALLOW, Mallow Mates	30g	102	427
PAMS			
Baby Choc Fish	25g	81	343
Chewy Pineapple Bites	25g	107	448
Chocolate Caramels	25g	125	525
Chocolate Peanuts	25g	142	595
Chocolate Raisins	25g	116	488
Fun Lollipops	10g	39	165
Gummy Party Mix	50g	168	705
Gummy Teddies	50g	168	705
Jelly Snakes	50g	179	750
Jumbo Jelly Beans	50g	193	808
Jumbo Mallows	50g	173	725
Licorice Allsorts	50g	194	815
Natural Licorice, Original	40g	133	560
Natural Licorice, Raspberry	40g	139	584
Soft Jubes	50g	172	723
Sour Party Mix	50g	167	702
PASCALL			
Chocolate Eclairs	25g	115	485
Curiously Strong	25g	99	418
Eskimos	25g	96	405

CONFECTIONERY

	QUANTITY	CALS	KJ
Fruit Burst	25g	95	400
Fruit Jubes	25g	88	370
Jaybees	25g	92	385
Jet Planes	25g	84	353
Licorice Allsorts	25g	97	410
Lolly Scramble	25g	99	415
Marshmallows	25g	82	345
Milk Bottles	25g	76	320
Mint Imperials	25g	101	423
Minties	25g	95	400
Party Pack	25g	85	358
Pineapple Lumps	25g	107	450
Spearmint Imperials	25g	101	423
Wine Gums	25g	85	358
RJ'S			
Licorice Allsorts	40g	156	654
Licorice Bullets	40g	165	688
Licorice Choc Logs	40g	153	640
Licorice Choc Twists	40g	153	640
Mango White Choc Log	40g	157	656
Mango White Choc Twists	40g	157	656
Natural Licorice	40g	136	572
Natural Licorice Log	40g	136	572
Natural Licorice Raspberry	40g	136	568
Raspberry Bullets	40g	165	692
Raspberry Choc Logs	40g	151	632
Raspberry Choc Twists	40g	151	632
SKITTLES			
Fruits	61g	250	1046
Sours	51g	200	836
Wild Berry	61g	250	1046
STARBURST			
Berry Berry Chews	25g	102	427
Fruitful Mix	25g	78	330
Gummi Fruits	25g	75	317

	QUANTITY	CALS	KJ
Mixed Berries	25g	81	339
Noughts & Crosses	25g	80	337
Party Mix	25g	77	326
Rattle Snakes	25g	77	325
Snakes & Ladders	25g	63	266
Sucks	each	45	192
THE NATURAL CONFECTIONERY CO.			
Fruity Chews	25g	23	100
Jellies			
Berry Bliss	25g	96	348
Dinosaurs	25g	82	345
Forbidden Fruit	25g	79	333
Jelly Babies	25g	81	343
Jelly Joiners	25g	82	344
Lolly Disguises	25g	76	321
Party Mix	25g	82	347
Smoothie Chews	25g	95	400
Snakes	25g	82	347
Sour Chews	25g	94	394
Strawberry & Cream Bliss	25g	81	340
Tangy Bliss	25g	84	355
Licorice Sticks	25g	87	368
Soft Jellies, Fruit Salad	25g	82	345
Sours, Squirms	25g	83	350
TIC TAC			
Fruit Adventure	100g	392	1665
Orange	100g	397	1685
Peppermint	100g	393	1669
Spearmint	100g	392	1672
Strawberry Fields	100g	391	1659
WERTHER'S ORIGINAL			
Caramel Creme	100g	405	1695
Classic Cream Candies	100g	424	1790
Classic Cream Candies, Sugar Free	100g	286	1200
Eclair	100g	457	1917

	QUANTITY	CALS	KJ
WHITTAKER'S			
K-Bars	each	102	429
Toffee Milks	each	49	207
WONKA			
Fabulicious Raspberry Twister	30g	114	480
Fabulicious Sherbert Fizz	30g	121	510

Crackers & Biscuits

	QUANTITY	CALS	KJ
ALISON'S PANTRY			
BBQ Rice Crackers	50g	271	1135
Chilli Rice Crackers	50g	270	1131
Digestive	50g	152	640
ARNOTT'S			
Cheds	23g	118	494
Cheeseboard	25g	113	475
Chocolate			
Butternut Snap	each	80	337
Caramel Crowns	each	75	317
Gaiety	each	71	298
Mint Slice	each	81	339
Scotch Finger	each	113	474
Country Cheese	3 biscuits	64	269
Creams			
Creamy Chocolate	each	73	309
Custard Cream	each	88	369
Kingston	each	66	279
Lemon Crisp	each	70	293
Monte Carlo	each	102	428
Orange Slice	each	71	301
Shortbread Cream	each	88	369
Cruskits			
Corn	2 biscuits	47	196
Light	2 biscuits	43	181
Rice	2 biscuits	45	189

	QUANTITY	CALS	KJ
Rye	2 biscuits	44	186
Digestive			
Dark Chocolate	each	81	339
Fruit & Milk Chocolate	each	81	339
Milk Chocolate	each	82	344
Family Plains			
Arno Shortbread	2 biscuits	118	497
Ginger Nut	2 biscuits	76	320
Malt 'O' Milk	3 biscuits	95	400
Marie	3 biscuits	108	452
Milk Arrowroot	3 biscuits	106	447
Milk Coffee	3 biscuits	110	461
Scotch Finger	each	87	366
Farmbake			
Butter Shortbread	2 biscuits	129	540
Chocolate Chip	2 biscuits	120	503
Chocolate Chip Fudge	2 biscuits	118	495
Crunchy Oat & Fruit	2 biscuits	117	493
Golden Crunch	2 biscuits	120	503
Orange Chocolate Chip	2 biscuits	115	482
Peanut Brownie	2 biscuits	122	513
Harvest Wheat	25g	120	505
Jatz, Clix	5 crackers	77	323
Kids			
Hundreds & Thousands	3 biscuits	68	287
Iced Animals	6 biscuits	145	610
Poppy & Sesame	25g	117	493
Salada			
Original	2 biscuits	119	500
Original Light	2 biscuits	136	570
Sesame Wheat	3 biscuits	189	376
Shapes			
Barbecue	25g	121	508
Cheddar	25g	119	500
Cheese & Bacon	25g	117	490

CRACKERS & BISCUITS

	QUANTITY	CALS	KJ
Chicken Crimpy	25g	117	490
Chicken Drumstick	25g	116	488
Pizza	25g	123	518
Sensations, Basil Pesto & Parmesan	20g	88	372
Sensations, Roasted Garlic & Parmesan	20g	89	374
Soundz, Chilli Supreme Pizza	25g	119	500
Soundz, Sweet & Sticky BBQ Ribs	25g	119	498
Soundz, Sweet Chilli & Sour Cream	25g	119	500
Supreme	20g	94	96
Tim Tam			
Chewy Caramel	each	96	405
Chocolicious Bites, Gooey Caramel	each	43	183
Chocolicious Bites, Original	each	47	198
Dark Choc	each	94	395
Double Coat	each	116	488
Original	each	95	399
Treat Pack, Adriana Zumbo, Choc Brownie	each	93	393
Treat Pack, Adriana Zumbo, Raspberry White Choc	each	95	399
Treat Pack, Adriana Zumbo, Salted Caramel	each	95	398
Treat Pack, Choc Mint	each	94	395
Treat Pack, Choc Orange	each	95	399
Treat Pack, Luscious Strawberry	each	95	399
Treat Pack, Turkish Delight	each	91	382
White	each	99	415
Tiny Teddy			
Choc Chip	25g	111	465
Chocolate	25g	111	468
Honey	25g	110	463
Vita-Weat			
9 Grains	4 crackers	86	364
Cracked Pepper	4 crackers	90	380
Original	4 crackers	90	378
Sesame	4 crackers	91	383

	QUANTITY	CALS	KJ
Vita-Weat Lunch Slices			
Mixed Grain & Toasted Sesame	2 crackers	154	646
Sesame Pumpkin & Quinoa	2 crackers	155	650
Soy Linseed & Sesame	2 crackers	154	646
Vita-Weat Rice Crackers			
Multigrain	22g	104	439
Plain	22g	102	430
Water Crackers, Original	6 biscuits	76	322
BELVITA			
Cranberry	4 biscuits	199	835
Crunchy Oats	4 biscuits	229	960
Fruit & Fibre	4 biscuits	224	940
Honey & Nut	4 biscuits	233	975
Milk & Cereals	4 biscuits	229	960
BUDGET			
Anzac Cookies	each	83	348
Assorted Family	11g	52	220
Choc Finger	25g	135	569
Choc Fudge Cookies	18g	81	342
Choc Tammy	18g	94	396
Chocolate Chippie	31g	146	614
Chocolate Cream	6g	30	128
Cream Cracker	41g	183	768
Cream Wafer	each	46	193
Fruit & Oat Cookies	18g	78	328
Gingernut	25g	114	478
Malt	34g	160	670
Milk Arrowroot	27g	119	500
Mini Creams			
Chocolate with Chocolate Cream	35g	159	669
Chocolate with Vanilla Cream	35g	161	676
Vanilla	35g	159	667
Nice Biscuits	9g	42	178
Peanut Brownie Cookies	18g	89	374
Plain Rounds	27g	128	539

CRACKERS & BISCUITS

	QUANTITY	CALS	KJ
Snacking Crackers	31g	145	610
Strawberry Cream	each	31	130
Super Rounds	20g	95	398
Vanilla Cream	6g	31	130
Vanilla Rounds	20g	105	440
Water Crackers	11g	46	194
CADBURY			
Fingers			
Chocolate	each	24	102
Honeycomb	each	23	99
Milk Chocolate	each	26	110
Freddo			
Chocolate	each	52	221
Vanilla	each	53	224
CERES ORGANICS			
Brown Rice Cakes			
No Added Salt	18g	71	298
Sea Salt	18g	68	286
Tamari	18g	69	290
Rice Crackers			
Black Sesame	12g	48	199
Sea Salt	12g	48	201
Tamari Soy	12g	47	200
COOKIE TIME			
Afghan Chocolate Chunk	each	494	2070
Apricot Chocolate Chunk	each	468	1960
Bite Size	3 biscuits	91	382
Chocolate Fix	each	310	1300
Gluten Free	each	311	1300
Nut & Chocolate Fix	each	287	1200
Original Chocolate Chunk	each	434	1820
Rookie, Triple Chocolate Chunk	each	120	503
Triple Chocolate Chunk	each	447	1870
White Chocolate Chunk	each	449	1880

	QUANTITY	CALS	KJ
ERNEST ADAMS			
Apricot Choc Cookies	14g	62	260
Chocolate Chip Cookies	14g	64	270
Double Chocolate Cookies	14g	64	270
Shortbread	14g	66	280
ETA			
Cravers			
Barbecue	20g	90	380
Chicken	20g	90	380
Pizza	20g	93	390
Smokey Bacon	20g	93	390
Spare Ribs	20g	93	390
FANTASTIC			
Crisp'ns			
Barbeque	25g	107	448
Cheese	25g	107	450
Original	25g	108	453
Salt & Balsamic Vinegar	25g	106	445
Sour Cream & Chives	25g	109	460
Sweet Chilli & Sour Cream	25g	108	455
Delites			
Cheddar Cheese	25g	111	468
Flame Grilled Barbeque	25g	108	453
Honey Soy Chicken	25g	110	463
Sour Cream & Chives	25g	110	463
Sweet Chilli & Sour Cream	25g	108	453
Traditional Chicken	25g	109	460
Vintage Cheddar & Red Onion	25g	111	465
Wood Fired Pizza	25g	103	435
Rice Crackers			
Barbeque	25g	100	420
Barbeque Chicken	25g	94	395
Cheddar Cheese	25g	106	445
Cheese	25g	109	458
Chicken	25g	101	425

CRACKERS & BISCUITS

	QUANTITY	CALS	KJ
French Onion & Cheese	25g	103	433
Oriental Teriyaki	25g	101	423
Original	25g	101	425
Salt & Vinegar	25g	94	395
Seaweed	25g	90	380
Sour Cream & Chives	25g	96	403
Sweet Chilli & Sour Cream	25g	103	433
GRIFFIN'S			
Afghans	each	81	340
Belgian Cremes	each	76	320
Cameo Cremes	each	77	325
Chit Chat	each	90	380
Choc Thins	each	36	153
Choc Thins, Jaffa	each	36	153
Chocolate Fingers	each	30	126
Cookie Bear Chocolate Chippies			
Mini	each	25	105
Mini – Choc Dipped	each	38	158
Original	each	44	186
Cookie Bear Hundreds & Thousands			
Mini	each	34	143
Original	each	50	210
Cookie Bear Partytime Wafers			
Mini	each	14	62
Original	each	47	200
Cookie Bear Shrewsbury	each	69	290
Cookie Bear Stripes	each	62	260
Digestive			
Fruit	each	57	240
Wheat	each	58	245
Dundee	2 biscuits	117	490
Fruitli Fingers, Apricot	each	42	176
Fruitli Fingers, Sultana	each	45	190
Gingernuts	each	54	230
Krispie			

	QUANTITY	CALS	KJ
Choc	each	66	280
Original	each	41	175
Lemon Treats	each	78	330
Macaroon	each	82	345
MallowPuffs			
Double Chocolate	each	88	370
Giant Original	each	274	1150
Original	each	88	370
Malt	each	36	152
Meal Mates			
Mini	25g	128	540
Mixed Vege	each	33	140
Original	each	33	140
Melting Moments	each	89	375
Milk Arrowroot	each	39	165
Mint Treat	each	87	365
Sensations, Peach	each	40	170
Shortbread	each	92	385
Snax, Original	each	20	84
Squiggles			
Candy	each	86	360
Hokey Pokey	each	88	370
Sultana Pasties	each	51	215
Swiss Cremes	each	63	265
Thin Table Water Crackers	each	43	180
Toffee Pops			
Butterscotch	each	81	340
Dark	each	80	335
Original	each	81	340
Wheaten			
Dark Chocolate	each	51	215
Milk Chocolate	each	51	215
Wines			
Round Wine	each	27	117
Super Wine	each	44	185

CRACKERS & BISCUITS

	QUANTITY	CALS	KJ
Vanilla Wine	each	78	330
HEALTHERIES			
Thick Corn Grain Wafers			
BBQ Chicken	each	40	127
Grains & Sunflower Seeds	each	16	70
Thick Rice Grain Wafers			
Mild Chilli	each	31	134
Smokey BBQ	each	30	128
Sour Cream & Chives	each	31	131
Whole Grain Rice	each	22	95
HOMEBRAND			
Anzac	each	104	436
Choco Chip Cookies	each	101	424
Chocolate Chip Cookies	2 biscuits	92	386
Creams	2 biscuits	97	407
Custard Cream	each	95	395
Fruit & Oat	each	94	394
Gingernut	2 biscuits	86	360
Malt	4 biscuits	143	600
Mint Slice	2 biscuits	160	663
Monty	2 biscuits	125	535
Rice Crackers, BBQ	25g	105	440
Rice Crackers, Plain	25g	103	435
Rice Crackers, Seaweed	25g	99	418
Round Tea	4 biscuits	119	500
Scotch Finger	each	86	360
Shortbread	each	86	360
Snax Crackers, Barbecue	25g	119	500
Snax Crackers, Chicken	25g	123	518
Strawberry Wafer	each	87	362
Traditional Cream Squares	2 crackers	81	340
Triple Choc	2 biscuits	182	763
Vanilla Creams	each	98	408
Vanilla Wafer	each	89	372
Wafers	each	87	364

	QUANTITY	CALS	KJ
Water Crackers, Cracked Pepper	4 crackers	65	226
Water Crackers, Traditional	4 crackers	54	228
HOTSHOTS			
Mr Munchies Cookies, My Little Pony	25g	119	500
Mr Munchies Cookies, Scooby Doo	25g	119	500
Mr Munchies Cookies, The Simpsons	25g	119	500
HUNTLEY & PALMERS			
10 Grain & Seeds Cracker Thins	4 crackers	109	460
Cheese Crackers, Cheese & Chives	3 crackers	107	450
Cheese Crackers, Tasty Cheese	4 crackers	107	450
Cream Crackers, Original	5 crackers	119	500
Cream Crackers, Reduced Fat	3 crackers	90	380
Litebread, Mixed Grain	each	24	100
Litebread, Original	each	24	100
Sesameal			
Classic 5 Grain	4 crackers	95	400
Olive Oil & Sea Salt	6 crackers	86	360
Original	4 crackers	95	400
Rosemary & Garlic	4 crackers	95	400
Somerset, Original	4 crackers	114	480
Wholegrain Crackers, 8 Grain	4 crackers	114	480
Wholegrain Crackers, Original Mixed Grain	4 crackers	109	460
MCVITIE'S			
Digestives			
Dark Chocolate	each	86	359
Milk Chocolate	each	86	359
NAIRNS			
Dark Chocolate Chip Oat Biscuits	each	44	183
Fine Milled Oat Cakes	each	36	151
Mixed Berry Oat Biscuits	each	43	182
Stem Ginger Oat Biscuits	each	43	180
OREO			
Chocolate	3 biscuits	142	596
Minis	12 biscuits	117	491
Original	3 biscuits	142	598

CRACKERS & BISCUITS

	QUANTITY	CALS	KJ
Peanut Butter & Chocolate Cream	3 biscuits	141	590
Strawberry	3 biscuits	141	590
ORGRAN			
Multigrain Crispibread with Quinoa	each	41	175
PAMS			
Rice Cakes			
Chocolate Topped	each	83	348
Dark Chocolate Orange Topped	each	80	338
Original	each	25	105
Sour Cream & Chives	each	31	132
Yoghurt Top	each	80	335
Rice Cracker Thins			
Original	25g	91	383
Sour Cream & Chives	25g	91	383
Tangy BBQ	25g	91	382
PECKISH			
Rice Crackers			
Cheddar Cheese	20g	91	382
Herb & Garlic	20g	90	378
Lime & Black Pepper	20g	87	368
Original	20g	89	373
Sea Salt & Vinegar	20g	89	374
Sweet Chilli	20g	88	372
Tangy BBQ	20g	86	360
Rice Snackers			
BBQ	25g	119	499
Cheese	25g	119	499
Pizza	25g	119	499
Sour Cream & Chives	25g	119	499
REAL FOODS			
Corn Thins			
Multigrain	each	23	97
Original	each	23	96
Sesame	each	23	96
Soy & Linseed	each	23	98

	QUANTITY	CALS	KJ
Rice Thins, Multigrain	each	24	100
RYVITA			
Crispbreads			
Multigrain	each	41	171
Original	each	35	146
Pumpkin Seeds & Oats	each	44	184
Sesame	each	37	154
SAKATA			
Rice Crackers			
Barbecue	25g	100	417
Plain	25g	99	416
Wholegrain Original	25g	99	414
SELECT			
Assorted Cream Selection	14g	67	281
Brown Rice Crackers, Cracked Pepper & Olive Oil	25g	104	438
Brown Rice Crackers, Multigrain	25g	102	428
Brown Rice Crackers, Sea Salt	25g	102	430
Butternut Chocolate Creams	14g	72	305
Chocolate Fingers	19g	17	72
Chocolate Mint Creme	16g	14	59
Chocolate Sandwich	19g	16	70
Garlic Crackers	20g	98	412
Lemon Creams	12g	55	232
Little Bears, Chocolate	25g	118	497
Little Bears, Honey	25g	107	450
Mallow Wheels	25g	28	119
Rocky Road Mallows	23g	25	105
Sea Salt Crackers	16g	12	53
Toffee Caramel	20g	97	410
Wheaten Biscuit, Original	10g	48	202
Wheaten Biscuit, Rosemary	10g	48	202
SIGNATURE RANGE			
Cheesy Snack Crackers	25g	121	510
Choc Thins	each	42	174

CRACKERS & BISCUITS

	QUANTITY	CALS	KJ
Chocolate Kisses	25g	102	425
Chocolate Wheaties	each	58	214
Ginger Kisses	each	103	430
Original Snack Crackers	25g	115	480
Rice Crackers			
Barbecue	25g	102	428
Plain	25g	99	415
Seaweed	25g	92	387
Wheat & Sesame Seed Crackers	25g	115	480
SUNRICE			
Rice & Corn Thin Rice Cakes, Original	100g	389	1630
Rice & Grain Squares			
Linseed	100g	365	1530
Quinoa	100g	353	1480
Seeds	100g	360	1510
Wild Rice	100g	358	1500
Thick Rice Cakes			
Lime & Cracked Pepper	100g	403	1690
Original	100g	389	1630
Salt & Balsamic Vinegar	100g	394	1650
Thin Rice Cakes			
Flame Grilled Barbecue	100g	399	1670
Original	100g	389	1630
Roast Chicken	100g	403	1690
Sweet Chilli & Sour Cream	100g	401	1680
Tasty Cheese	100g	402	1680
WATERTHINS			
Bagelettes, Original	25g	114	478
Cheese Twists, Classic Cheddar	each	42	178
Corn Wafer Thins	20g	85	356
Fine Wafer Crackers	6 crackers	39	165
Fine Wafer Crackers, Sesame	6 crackers	40	168
WELLABY'S			
Crackers, Classic Cheese	30g	131	552
Hummus Chips, Kalamata Olive	30g	126	529

	QUANTITY	CALS	KJ
Lentils Chips, Rosemary	30g	120	506

Dairy & Soy Products

Butter & Margarine

ALFA ONE

	QUANTITY	CALS	KJ
Cholestrol Lowering	100g	720	3010
Rice Bran Oil Spread	100g	668	2800
Rice Bran Oil Spread, Lite	100g	502	2100
ALPINE, Butter	100g	724	3030
ANCHOR			
Blue Dairy Blend	10g	62	261
Butter	10g	72	303
Calcit	10g	53	225
Lite Dairy Blend	10g	53	225
Trim Dairy Blend	10g	35	148
BUDGET, Table Spread	10g	21	89
CONSTANTINA, Garlic Spread	100g	660	2761
COUNTRY SOFT			
Light	100g	459	1930
Original	100g	610	2550
FLORA			
Buttery	10g	62	261
Canola	10g	57	242
Light	10g	42	177
Original	10g	58	242
Pro-activ			
Buttery	10g	57	241
Light	10g	35	150
Olive	10g	43	180
Original	10g	56	238
Ultra Light	10g	21	90
Salt Reduced	10g	57	242
Ultra Light	10g	22	96

DAIRY & SOY PRODUCTS

	QUANTITY	CALS	KJ
GOLD'N CANOLA			
Lite	10g	40	170
Original	10g	57	240
HOMEBRAND, Table Spread	100g	573	2400
LEWIS ROAD CREAMERY			
Artisan	100g	748	3130
Premium	100g	728	3050
LURPAK			
Lighter Spreadable Slightly Salted	100g	544	2994
Spreadable Slightly Salted	100g	728	2237
MAINLAND, Butter			
Natural	100g	740	3090
Semi-soft	100g	725	3030
MEADOWLEA			
Canola	10g	57	240
Cook & Bake Buttery, Original	10g	62	260
Cook & Bake Buttery, Unsalted	10g	62	260
Heart Plus Lite	10g	41	175
Lite	10g	43	180
Original	10g	57	240
Salt Reduced	10g	57	240
OLIVANI			
Avocado	10g	49	206
Olive Oil	10g	57	240
Olive Oil Lite	10g	24	102
PAMS			
Original	5g	48	205
SUNRISE, Table Spread	10g	48	205
TARARUA			
Butter	100g	730	3040
Super-soft	100g	633	2650
Super-soft, Lite	100g	544	2280
WEIGHT WATCHERS, Canola Spread	100g	406	1700

	QUANTITY	CALS	KJ
Cheese			
Cottage Cheese			
Lite	45g	38	160
Standard	25g	48	203
Cream Cheese			
Lite	25g	60	249
Standard	25g	93	384
Mascarpone	20g	90	376
Ricotta	20g	35	145
ANCHOR			
Colby	25g	100	420
Edam	25g	87	365
Mild	25g	105	440
Tasty	25g	105	440
BEGA, Stringers, Original	each	59	250
BOUTON D'OR			
Blue Vein	100g	338	1415
Double Cream Camembert	100g	406	1700
Feta			
Basil Pesto	100g	242	1015
Garlic & Cumin	100g	240	1005
Goat Feta	100g	236	990
Plain	100g	239	1000
Reduced Salt	100g	239	1000
Sundried Tomato	100g	236	990
Mini Brie	100g	375	1570
BUDGET, Cheese Slices	21g	52	219
CASTELLO			
Blue	100g	430	1780
White	100g	410	1690
DAIRYWORKS			
Blocks			
Colby	20g	79	334
Edam	20g	69	292
Extreme Tasty	20g	85	358

DAIRY & SOY PRODUCTS

	QUANTITY	CALS	KJ
Gouda	20g	74	310
Mozzarella	20g	62	260
Tasty	20g	85	358
Cheese & Crackers			
Colby	30g	119	501
Edam	30g	107	448
Tasty	50g	209	877
Cheese Slices			
Colby	20g	79	334
Edam	20g	69	292
Gouda	20g	74	310
Swiss	20g	73	306
Tasty	20g	85	358
Cheese Sticks	20g	69	292
Mini Slices			
Edam	6g	21	88
Gouda	6g	22	93
Tasty	6g	25	107
Parmesan Powder	20g	91	382
Parmesan Wedge	20g	73	306
GALAXY			
Blue Vein	100g	332	1390
Creamy Feta	100g	203	853
Mozzarella	100g	288	1206
HOMEBRAND			
Cheese Slices	100g	292	1220
Colby	100g	400	1670
Edam	100g	349	1460
Mild	100g	423	1770
Tasty	100g	423	1770
KAPITI			
Aorangi	20g	77	324
Awa Blue	20g	66	280
Cumin Seed Gouda	20g	74	310
Emmental	20g	78	328

	QUANTITY	CALS	KJ
Kahikatea Camembert	20g	77	324
Kahurangi Creamy Blue	20g	90	380
Kanuka Waxed Havarti	20g	82	344
Karu	20g	68	288
Kikorangi	20g	87	368
Pakari Aged Cheddar	20g	84	354
Pakari Smoked Cheddar	20g	84	355
Port Wine Cheddar	20g	84	354
Ramara	20g	64	270
Smoked Havarti	20g	82	344
Tuteremoana Cheddar	20g	84	354
LEMNOS			
Fetta			
Full Cream	30g	95	399
Goat's Milk	30g	77	322
Organic Full Cream	30g	92	382
Organic Reduced Fat	30g	79	330
Reduced Fat	30g	89	370
Reduced Fat Smooth	30g	14	60
Sheep's Milk	30g	82	342
Smooth	25g	63	264
Goat's Cheese	20g	53	222
Haloumi			
Organic	30g	86	360
Original	30g	102	426
Reduced Salt	30g	101	425
With Antipasto	30g	85	356
With Chilli	30g	87	362
MAINLAND			
Colby	25g	98	412
Edam	25g	86	360
Egmont	25g	105	440
Epicure	25g	106	445
Mild	25g	105	440
Noble	25g	89	375

DAIRY & SOY PRODUCTS

	QUANTITY	CALS	KJ
Parmesan	25g	85	357
Smoked	25g	107	450
Swiss	25g	98	410
Tasty	25g	106	445
Tasty Light	25g	80	337
Vegetarian Edam	25g	86	360
Vintage	25g	106	445
ORNELLE			
Brie	100g	372	1560
Camembert	100g	275	1570
Double Cream Brie	100g	406	1700
Feta	100g	239	1000
Parmesan	100g	348	1460
PAMS			
Colby Slices	20g	64	269
Edam Slices	20g	64	269
PERFECT ITALIANO			
Parmesan	10g	38	162
Pizza Plus	25g	85	358
PUHOI VALLEY			
40 Acre Basil Pesto Cow Feta	30g	232	970
40 Acre Cow Feta	30g	230	960
Chilli & Kaffir Layered Havarti	30g	400	1670
Distinction Blue Cheese	100g	416	1740
Fresh Goat Cheese	30g	230	960
Intrepid Gorgonzola Style Blue	30g	352	1470
Mascarpone	30g	450	1880
Mini Creamy Blue	70g	402	1680
Mini Double Cream Camembert	60g	407	1700
Mini Peppered Havarti	70g	400	1670
Mini Single Cream Brie	60g	383	1600
Mini Smokey Gouda	70g	371	1550
Oakdale Clode Camembert	30g	376	1570
Old Barn Brie	30g	276	1570
Parmesan Wedge	30g	364	1520

	QUANTITY	CALS	KJ
Riverside Red	30g	416	1740
Rolling Pastures Triple Cream Brie	30g	417	1741
Secret Blue Brie	30g	390	1630
Stable Door Parmesan	21g	471	1970
Tarragon & Garlic Havarti	30g	400	1670
View Goat Feta	30g	234	980
Winding Track Double Cream Brie	30g	407	1700
SIGNATURE RANGE			
Blocks			
Colby	100g	408	1710
Edam	100g	351	1470
Mild	100g	432	1810
Tasty	100g	432	1810
Brie, Double Cream	25g	101	422
Classic Blue Vein	25g	100	422
Classic Camembert	25g	90	420
Classic Creamy Blue	25g	114	375
Slices			
Colby	100g	309	1290
Edam	100g	322	1346
Tasty	100g	311	1300
Traditional Brie	25g	87	363
Cream			
Coconut Cream, Lite	100mL	87	364
Coconut Cream, Standard	100mL	200	837
Sour Cream, Lite	100mL	152	636
Sour Cream, Standard	100mL	236	987
ALPRO, Soya Single	100g	169	698
ANCHOR			
Fresh Cream	100mL	348	1456
Longlife Cream	100mL	335	1410
Thickened Cream	100mL	385	1608
HOMEBRAND, Fresh Cream	100mL	331	1385
LEWIS ROAD CREAMERY			
Double Cream	100mL	449	1880

DAIRY & SOY PRODUCTS

	QUANTITY	CALS	KJ
Single Cream	100mL	338	1418
MEADOW FRESH, Fresh Cream	100mL	330	1385
PAMS, Cream	100mL	106	447
SELECT			
Whipped Cream, Light	100g	229	961
Whipped Cream, Regular	100g	293	1230
Milk Drinks			
ANCHOR			
CalciYum Singles			
Banana	100mL	59	249
Caramel	100mL	59	249
Chocolate	100mL	59	348
Strawberry	100mL	59	247
FOR EVERYONE			
Banana	100mL	68	285
Chocolate	100mL	71	300
Strawberry	100mL	69	290
MAMMOTH ICED COFFEE			
Mocha	100mL	67	280
Original	100mL	63	260
Strong	100mL	63	260
MEADOW FRESH			
Banana	100mL	68	287
Calci Strong, Banana	100mL	68	287
Calci Strong, Chocolate	100mL	71	299
Calci Strong, Strawberry	100mL	68	287
Chocolate	100mL	71	299
Drinking Yoghurt, all flavours	100mL	65	275
Strawberry	100mL	68	287
NIPPY'S			
Iced Chocolate	100mL	63	267
Iced Coffee	100mL	59	251
Iced Mocha	100mL	61	259
Iced Vanilla	100mL	64	271

	QUANTITY	CALS	KJ
PRIMO			
Banana, Lime & Strawberry Flavours	100mL	62	260
Chocolate	100mL	67	280
SANITARIUM			
Up & Go			
Banana	350mL	277	1180
Choc Ice	350mL	277	1150
Energize Chocolate	350mL	308	1280
Energize Iced Coffee	350mL	291	1210
Energize Vanilla	350mL	294	1230
Strawberry	350mL	277	1160
Vanilla Ice	350mL	277	1150
Vive Chocolate	250mL	167	695
Vive Vanilla	250mL	168	700
V, Iced Coffee	100mL	70	294
WAVE			
Chocolate	600mL	489	2050
Strawberry	600mL	480	2010
Milk & Substitutes			
A2 MILK	100mL	63	260
ANCHOR			
Blue	100mL	62	260
Calci+	100mL	46	195
Lite	100mL	46	194
Mega	100mL	58	243
Silver Top	100mL	69	290
Trim	100mL	40	168
North Island	100mL	37	153
South Island	100mL	40	167
Zero Lacto			
Blue	100mL	62	260
Trim	100mL	62	260
DELAMERE			
Semi-skimmed Goats Milk	100mL	45	190
Whole Goats Milk	100mL	62	257

DAIRY & SOY PRODUCTS

	QUANTITY	CALS	KJ
FREEDOM FOODS			
Rice Milk	100mL	65	212
Soy Milk, Original	100mL	56	234
HOMEBRAND			
Full Cream UHT Milk	100mL	64	268
Lite	100mL	47	200
Rice Milk	100mL	58	245
Soy Drink	100mL	71	300
Standard	100mL	60	255
Trim	100mL	40	170
LEWIS ROAD CREAMERY			
Calcium Enriched, Low Fat	100mL	43	184
Homogenised	100mL	70	295
Non-Homogenised	100mL	70	295
LIDDELLS, Lactose Free, Low Fat	100mL	42	175
MACRO			
Full Cream Milk UHT	100mL	63	262
Light Milk UHT	100mL	45	190
Light Soy Drink	100mL	51	215
Rice Milk	100mL	65	275
Soy Drink	100mL	74	311
MEADOW FRESH			
Enriched			
Calci Strong, Lite	100mL	56	235
Calci Strong, Original	100mL	60	255
Calci Trim	100mL	45	190
Everyday			
Farmhouse	100mL	66	280
Lite	100mL	47	200
Organic Original	100mL	59	250
Original	100mL	60	255
Trim	100mL	40	170
PAMS			
Calci Smart	100mL	92	385
Regular Rice Milk	100mL	51	216

	QUANTITY	CALS	KJ
Slim	100mL	47	200
Standard	100mL	62	260
Slim	100mL	34	145
Standard	100mL	64	268
UHT Milk			
Slim	100mL	34	145
Standard	100mL	64	268
RICE DREAM, Original	100mL	49	209
SELECT			
Calci-Choice	100mL	45	190
Full Cream	100mL	67	281
SIGNATURE RANGE			
Lite	100mL	48	200
Organic Rice Milk	100mL	61	255
Organic Soy	100mL	41	170
Organic Soy, Lite	100mL	50	210
Standard	100mL	66	280
Trim	100mL	52	220
SO GOOD			
Almond & Coconut	100mL	27	113
Almond Milk	100mL	31	130
Almond Milk, Unsweetened	100mL	17	71
Chocolate Bliss	100mL	60	250
Essential UHT	100mL	53	221
Lite	100mL	41	171
Lite UHT	100mL	41	171
Milky	100mL	48	198
Regular	100mL	65	273
Regular UHT	100mL	65	273
UHT Rice Milk	100mL	51	214
Vanilla Bliss	100mL	60	250
SUN LATTE, Milk	100mL	44	185
TARARUA, Cultured Buttermilk	100g	38	160
VITASOY			
Calci-plus Soymilk	100mL	64	270

DAIRY & SOY PRODUCTS

	QUANTITY	CALS	KJ
Oatmilk Bone Essentials	100mL	61	25
Oatmilk Honey Delight	100mL	71	299
Original Soymilk	100mL	64	269
Reduced Fat	100mL	49	208
Ricemilk Original	100mL	50	209
Ricemilk Protein Enriched	100mL	55	231
Soy Milky	100mL	53	220
Soy Milky, Lite	100mL	38	159
Unsweetened Soy Milk	100mL	16	68
Vanilla	100mL	54	224
VitaGo			
Banana & Honey	100mL	80	334
Chocolate	100mL	80	334
Vitality Soymilk	100mL	44	186
Yoghurt			
ANCHOR			
CalciYum			
Banana	100g	82	343
Caramel	100g	82	344
Chocolate Banana	100g	82	343
Chocolate, Milk Chocolate	100g	83	347
Cookie & Cream	100g	82	343
Strawberry	100g	82	343
Wicked Chocolate	100g	83	346
BIOFARM ORGANIC			
Acidophilus	100mL	68	288
Bush Honey	100mL	87	367
Low Fat	100mL	35	149
CYCLOPS			
Banana	100g	75	317
Blueberry	100g	104	436
Boysenberry	100g	66	280
Chocolate	100g	163	683
Chocolate Velvet	100g	163	683
Citrus	100g	75	316

	QUANTITY	CALS	KJ
Coffee	100g	132	553
Lemon Honey	100g	129	542
Low Fat	100g	58	244
Low Fat Greek	100g	86	360
Raspberry	100g	69	291
Strawberry	100g	70	294
Thick & Creamy	100g	118	496
Walnut & Honey	100g	112	471
DE WINKEL, Plain Unsweetened	100g	50	211
EASIYO YOGURT BASE			
Everyday Range			
Apricot	100g	102	427
Banana	100g	105	437
Boysenberry	100g	96	403
Caramel	100g	113	471
Forest Fruits	100g	96	402
Greek Style	100g	82	344
Lemon	100g	95	399
Mango	100g	101	423
Natural	100g	68	283
Peach	100g	103	429
Raspberry	100g	96	400
Strawberry	100g	104	434
Summer Fruits	100g	104	433
Sweet Greek	100g	107	447
Toffee	100g	107	448
Vanilla	100g	197	433
Gourmet Range			
Blueberries & Cream	100g	106	443
Cranberries & Bits	100g	108	453
Custard Style	100g	100	419
Greek & Coconut Bits	100g	113	472
Greek & Honey	100g	98	409
Mixed Berry & Bits	100g	104	435
Peaches & Cream	100g	110	461

DAIRY & SOY PRODUCTS

	QUANTITY	CALS	KJ
Raspberries & Cream	100g	108	451
Strawberries & Cream	100g	111	466
Vanilla Peach & Bits	100g	103	432
Nutrition Range			
Biolife Organic, Unsweetened	100g	70	294
Low Fat Greek	100g	66	275
Low Fat Mango	100g	76	319
Low Fat Strawberry	100g	74	309
Low Fat Sweet Vanilla	100g	76	319
Reduced Fat, Unsweetened	100g	62	257
Skimmers, Unsweetened	100g	50	206
FRESH 'N FRUITY			
Greek Style			
Low Fat	100g	74	310
Natural	100g	123	514
Lite			
Apricot	100g	51	211
Apricot Crumble	100g	49	203
Apricot, Peach & Pear	100g	50	211
Berries & Cherries	100g	51	213
Mango Passion	100g	62	261
Peach Passion	100g	51	212
Pineapple Passion	100g	62	261
Simply Strawberry	100g	41	172
Strawberry	100g	49	203
Vanilla Dream	100g	43	178
Wildly Berry	100g	49	206
Regular			
Apple Crumble	100g	94	395
Apricot	100g	89	371
Apricot & Custard	100g	105	440
Apricot & Vanilla	100g	105	437
Banana, Pear & Custard	100g	98	409
Berries & Cherries	100g	97	407
Berries & Cream	100g	96	400

	QUANTITY	CALS	KJ
Berry Combo	100g	95	398
Blackberry & Cream	100g	100	417
Boysenberry & Cream	100g	96	400
Dreamy Lemon	100g	106	445
Fruit of the Forest	100g	98	410
Mango, Apricot & Vanilla	100g	104	436
Mango & Passionfruit	100g	100	419
Mango & Pineapple	100g	100	419
Natural	100g	87	363
Passion Cheesecake	100g	93	387
Passion Pineapple	100g	96	399
Peach & Passionfruit	100g	95	398
Peaches & Cream	100g	95	398
Raspberry & Cream	100g	102	425
Rhubarb & Custard	100g	100	418
Simply Apricot	100g	88	369
Simply Strawberry	100g	91	379
Strawberries & Cream	100g	93	390
Vanilla Bean	100g	108	451
HANSELLS YOGHURT BASE			
BioHealth			
Prebiotic Greek Style	100g	101	420
Vanilla, Peach & Honey	100g	77	323
Classic, Natural	100g	69	287
Lite			
Natural	100g	52	217
Natural Greek Style	100g	74	310
Passionfruit	100g	70	294
Low Lactose, Natural	100g	58	243
Super Fruits with Bits, Goji & Red Superberries	100g	114	475
Thick & Creamy			
Greek & Coconut	100g	115	481
Greek & Honey	100g	102	427
Mango Passion	100g	104	436

DAIRY & SOY PRODUCTS

	QUANTITY	CALS	KJ
Natural Greek Style	100g	108	451
Strawberry	100g	103	430
MEADOW FRESH			
Live Lite, all flavours	100mL	75	315
Pre-Bio			
Black Cherry & Vanilla	100mL	120	505
Blackberry, Blueberry & Vanilla	100mL	118	495
Boysenberry, Cranberry & Blueberry	100mL	113	475
Caramelised Pear	100mL	119	500
Fig & Honey	100mL	119	500
French Vanilla	100mL	119	500
Maple Vanilla	100mL	119	500
Pear, Blackcurrant & Acai	100mL	118	495
Rhubarb with a Hint of Ginger	100mL	117	490
Strawberry & Pomegranate	100mL	120	505
Strawberry & Vanilla	100mL	120	505
Vanilla Bean	100mL	119	500
Regular			
Apple & Cinnamon Custard	100mL	95	400
Apricot	100mL	86	360
Apricot, Orange & Passion	100mL	86	360
Banana Custard	100mL	93	390
Blackberry	100mL	86	360
Boysenberry	100mL	86	360
Boysenberry & Cream	100mL	86	360
Mango & Passion	100mL	90	380
Mixed Berries	100mL	83	350
Natural Sweetened	100mL	78	330
Passion Peach	100mL	90	380
Raspberry & Cream	100mL	86	360
Strawberry	100mL	88	370
Strawberry & Cream	100mL	88	370
Smooth			
Mixed Berries	100mL	82	345
Strawberry	100mL	82	345

	QUANTITY	CALS	KJ
Thick & Creamy			
Blackberry & Cream	100mL	109	460
French Vanilla	100mL	109	460
Juicy Orange	100mL	107	450
Mango Papaya Passion	100mL	137	575
Pineapple & Coconut	100mL	136	570
Plump Apricot	100mL	105	440
Raspberry & Cream	100mL	105	440
Strawberry & Cream	100mL	105	440
Strawberry & Pomegranate	100mL	137	575
Vanilla Bean	100mL	109	460
Vanilla Spice	100mL	109	460
Zesty Lemon	100mL	107	450
NATURALEA, Plain Unsweetened	100g	57	240
PIAKO			
Apricot & Peach	100g	140	587
Blackcurrant Cranberry	100g	122	509
Lemon Curd	100g	125	524
Mango	100g	133	557
Mixed Berry	100g	130	545
Natural Sweetened	100g	131	547
Passionfruit	100g	130	542
Peach Orange	100g	123	514
Strawberry Honey	100g	121	506
Vanilla Bean	100g	140	587
PUHOI VALLEY			
Apricot & Honey	150g	136	570
Divine Berries	150g	136	570
Fabulous Feijoa	150g	141	590
Greek Style	150g	138	575
Heavenly Rhubarb	150g	139	580
Lemon Delicious	150g	170	710
Luscious Nectarine	150g	141	590
Orange Citrus	150g	139	580
Raspberry Dream	150g	144	600

DAIRY & SOY PRODUCTS

	QUANTITY	CALS	KJ
SLIMMER'S CHOICE, Low Fat	100g	55	231
SYMBIO			
Apricot & Mango	100g	87	356
Mixed Berry	100g	77	321
Natural Unsweetened	100g	56	236
Passionfruit	100g	81	339
Pouring Yoghurt			
Strawberry	100g	67	281
Vanilla	100g	62	260
Rhubarb	100g	80	337
Vanilla Bean	100g	82	339
Wholegrains			
Apricot	100g	85	356
Blueberry	100g	87	366
THE COLLECTIVE			
Gourmet Yoghurt			
Apple Crumble	100g	138	581
Black Plum	100g	137	574
Bloody Ovarige	100g	135	567
Coconuts	100g	137	574
Luscious Lemon	100g	138	579
Mango	100g	134	564
Natural	100g	105	440
Passionfruit	100g	138	580
Peach	100g	133	558
Raspberry Choccy	100g	108	455
Rhubarb & Strawberry	100g	136	571
Russian Fudge	100g	145	610
Straight Up	100g	102	430
Pourable Yoghurt			
Boys'nberry	100mL	87	366
Tummy Love	100mL	50	210
Yummy Runny Yoghurt	100mL	88	369
Suckies Pouches			
Blueberry	100g	89	373

	QUANTITY	CALS	KJ
Honeycomb	100g	94	395
Nommy Banana	100g	100	420
Peach & Apricot	100g	89	374
Sassy Strawberry	100g	104	438
Suckies Tubes			
Bonkers 4 Bananas	100g	105	441
Bouncing Berries	100g	103	433
Sassy Strawberry	100g	100	419
WEIGHT WATCHERS, Natural	100g	82	344
YOPLAIT			
Delite			
Blackberry	100g	75	309
Citrus	100g	84	353
Mixed Berry	100g	72	302
Peach & Mango	100g	69	291
Raspberry	100g	75	314
Strawberry	100g	75	314
Vanilla	100g	75	315
Elivaé			
Berry Mixed	100g	81	341
Fig & Honey	100g	85	358
Peach & Apricot	100g	85	357
Vanilla	100g	84	353
Greek Style, Honey	100g	111	466
Lite Natural	100g	88	370
Natural	100g	111	467
Petit Miam			
Apricot	100g	135	568
Banana	100g	140	583
Peach	100g	137	575
Raspberry	100g	134	559
Strawberry	100g	134	561
Vanilla	100g	133	559
Regular			
Apple & Cinnamon	100g	88	370

DAIRY & SOY PRODUCTS/DESSERTS

	QUANTITY	CALS	KJ
Blackberry	100g	89	375
Citrus	100g	100	419
Citrus Burst	100g	100	421
Citrus Twist	100g	95	401
Lemon	100g	98	413
Mixed Berry	100g	89	375
Passionfruit	100g	91	384
Peach & Mango	100g	85	358
Raspberry	100g	90	380
Strawberry	100g	90	380
Vanilla	100g	91	381
Seriously Smooth			
Banana Custard	100g	75	313
Blueberry	100g	76	317
Passionfruit	100g	75	316
Peach	100g	76	317
Strawberry	100g	76	319
Vanilla	100g	75	314
Vanilla Custard	100g	74	313
Vigueur			
Caramel Choc	100g	113	475
Chocolate Eclair	100g	113	476
Chocolate Mudcake	100g	113	475
Classic Choc	100g	114	477
Yogo Xtreme Chocolate	100g	87	364
Yoplus			
Natural	100g	71	297
Trim	100g	50	211

Desserts

AUNT BETTY'S			
Creamy Rice			
Chocolate	100g	116	485
Vanilla	100g	102	429

	QUANTITY	CALS	KJ
Vanilla with Peach	100g	89	372
Healthy De-lites, Sticky Date	100g	269	1130
Ready to Eat Custard	100g	91	381
Saucy Centre Puddings			
Chocolate	100g	388	1630
Lemon	100g	360	1510
Steamed Puddings			
Chocolate	100g	306	1320
Dark Chocolate	100g	291	1220
Golden Fruit	100g	294	1230
Golden Syrup	100g	309	1290
Gooey Caramel	100g	289	1210
CADBURY, Ice Cream			
Caramello	100g	211	883
Dairy Milk Chip	100g	232	971
Triple Chocolate	100g	217	910
CROFTERS			
Cheesecake			
Boysenberry	100g	286	1190
Passionfruit	100g	296	1240
Strawberry	100g	294	1230
White Chocolate & Raspberry Bavarian	100g	291	1210
DOLE			
Fruit & Custard			
Mango	100g	94	392
Peach	100g	92	382
Fruit & Jelly, Peach	100g	93	389
GREGG'S			
Crumble Mix	100g	412	1720
Instant Desserts, all flavours	100g	369	1540
Jelly, all flavours	100g	58	242
Rich Chocolate Mousse	100g	49	624
HANSELLS			
Chocolate Mousse	100mL	90	378
Crème Brulée	100mL	333	1390

DESERTS

	QUANTITY	CALS	KJ
HOMEBRAND			
Apple Pie	100g	243	1020
Chocolate Bavarian	100g	303	1270
Creamed Rice	100g	111	462
Custard Powder	100g	304	270
Instant Desserts			
Butterscotch Crunch	100g	385	1610
Choc-a-lot with Chocolate Chips	100g	395	1650
Strawberry Sponge Cheesecake	100g	386	1610
Vanilla Crème	100g	386	1610
Strawberry Cheesecake	100g	270	1130
JUICIES			
Organic Apple	each	47	197
Tropical	each	44	188
Wildberry	each	43	182
KAPITI			
Ice Cream			
Gingernut	100mL	272	1140
Triple Chocolate	100mL	261	1090
Vanilla Bean	100mL	259	1080
White Chocolate & Raspberry	100mL	220	1060
Sorbet			
Lemon	100mL	69	290
Lime	100mL	84	354
Raspberry	100mL	63	265
KILLINCHY GOLD			
Ice Cream			
Boysenberry Cheesecake	100g	240	1010
Chocolate Fudge Brownie	100g	276	1120
Gold Rock Hokey Pokey	100g	245	1030
Maple Syrup & Walnuts	100g	250	1050
Pure Vanilla	100g	230	970
Salted Caramel & Cashew	100g	255	1070

	QUANTITY	CALS	KJ
KIWI			
Ice Cream			
Cappuccino Fudge	100g	204	855
Chocolate	100g	146	612
Cookies	100g	214	896
French Vanilla	100g	192	804
Marshmallow Strawberry	100g	190	800
Neopolitan	100g	195	816
Strawberry	100g	193	809
Tropical	100g	190	797
Vanilla	100g	201	843
Vanilla, Low Fat	100g	197	620
MINOO			
Gelato, Chocolate	100g	200	837
Sorbet			
Lemon	100g	117	489
Wildberry	100g	95	395
MÖVENPICK			
Ice Cream			
Caramelita	100g	260	1089
Crème Brûlée	100g	239	999
Maple Walnut	100g	263	1102
Swiss Chocolate	100g	303	1263
Tiramisu	100g	270	1131
Vanilla Dream	100g	257	1072
NANNA'S			
Original Waffles	100g	255	1070
Snack Pies			
Apple	100g	333	1000
Apricot	100g	265	1170
Blackberry & Apple	100g	310	1240
NEW ZEALAND NATURAL			
Ice Cream			
Chocolate Hokey Pokey	100g	260	1090
White Chocolate & Raspberry	100g	240	1010

DESSERTS

	QUANTITY	CALS	KJ
Sorbet			
Lemon Lime Sorbet	100g	125	520
Mango Sorbet	100g	130	550
OMAHA ORGANIC BERRIES			
Ice Cream			
Double Chocolate	100g	270	1130
Macadamia Nut & Honey	100g	279	1170
Peppermint Chip	100g	262	1100
Vanilla	100g	246	1030
PAMS			
Apple & Rhubarb Pie	100g	215	902
Apple Crumble Blossoms	100g	69	292
Boysenberry Cheesecake	100g	315	1320
Chocolate Chiplara Cookie Cakes	100g	105	441
Chocolate Mousse	100g	460	1930
Cream Puffs	100g	325	1360
Creamed Rice			
Lite Vanilla	100g	92	385
Vanilla	100g	112	470
Eclairs	100g	356	490
Fiesta			
Chocolate	100g	184	772
Strawberry	100g	185	775
Gateau			
Double Chocolate	100g	267	1120
Sweet Strawberry	100g	250	1050
Ice Cream			
Classic Vanilla	100g	160	670
Crushed Cookies	100g	185	776
Do The Hokey Pokey	100g	216	740
Très French Vanilla	100g	160	671
Instant Desserts	100g	379	1590
Banana	100g	384	1610
Butterscotch	100g	384	1610
Chocolate	100g	380	1590

	QUANTITY	CALS	KJ
Chocolate Fudge	100g	380	1590
Raspberry	100g	384	1610
Strawberry	100g	384	1610
Vanilla	100g	284	1610
Jelly			
Lemon	100g	59	249
Lime	100g	59	250
Orange	100g	59	250
Raspberry	100g	59	251
Strawberry	100g	59	249
Mini Eclairs	100g	343	1438
Passionfruit Cheesecake	100g	310	1300
Strawberry Cheesecake	100g	308	1290
Traditional Apple Pie	100g	215	902
RUSH MUNRO'S			
Ice Cream			
Cookies & Cream	100g	232	975
Hokey Pokey	100g	235	985
Mochaccino	100g	213	895
Passionfruit	100g	203	852
Vanilla Bean	100g	213	918
SARA LEE			
Apple Crumble	100g	277	1160
Apple Strudel	100g	313	1310
Belgian Chocolate Pudding	100g	380	1590
Caramel Chocolate Bavarian	100g	341	1430
Carrot Cake	100g	365	1530
Cheesecake			
Chocolate	100g	358	1500
Chocolate Swirl Bavarian	100g	329	1380
Cookies & Cream Bavarian	100g	344	1440
French Cream	100g	372	1560
Mixed Berry	100g	327	1370
Strawberry	100g	320	1340
Chocolate Cake	100g	380	1590

DESSERTS

	QUANTITY	CALS	KJ
Chocolate Pudding	100g	303	1270
Classic Apple Pie	100g	317	1330
Danish			
Apricot	each	241	1011
Blueberry	each	185	776
Dish Pie			
Apple & Berry Pie	100g	284	1190
Apple Crumble	100g	289	1210
Entertainer Bavarian Triple Chocolate	100g	365	1530
Sticky Date Pudding	100g	336	1410
Tiramisu	100g	346	1450
SIGNATURE RANGE			
Creamed Rice			
Chocolate	100g	120	505
Vanilla	100g	91	380
Ice Cream			
Boysenberry Ripple	100g	198	833
Chocolate	100g	203	854
Chocolate Éclair	100g	215	901
French Vanilla	100g	202	848
Hokey Pokey	100g	214	900
Neopolitan	100g	203	850
Vanilla	100g	202	848
SO GOOD			
Frozen Dessert			
Chocolate Bliss	100g	146	610
Vanilla Bliss	100g	151	630
STREETS			
Bubble O Bill	each	149	622
Calippo			
Cola Lemonade	each	89	374
Raspberry Pineapple	each	89	376
Cookie Crumble	each	233	979
Cornetto			
Classic Supreme Chocolate	each	204	856

	QUANTITY	CALS	KJ
Enigma Vanilla & Chocolate	each	259	1085
Enigma Vanilla & Raspberry	each	475	988
Vanilla Choc Nut	each	211	887
Magnum			
Almond	each	399	1357
Chocolate Truffle	each	282	1179
Classic	each	282	1181
Ego Caramel	each	341	1426
Gold	each	379	1588
Honeycomb Crunch	each	310	1299
Peppermint	each	275	1151
Pink	each	298	1209
Strawberry White Crumble	each	320	1338
Paddle Pop			
Chocolate	each	79	330
Cyclone	each	90	376
Icy Twist	each	63	266
Rainbow	each	107	449
Splice, Pine Lime	each	83	351
Viennetta, Vanilla	100g	261	1094
TIP TOP			
Crammed			
Berry Choc Forest	100g	259	1080
Choc Eruption	100g	285	1180
Jamming Cream Donut	100g	227	950
Favourites			
Choc Bar	each	285	1190
Eskimo Pie	each	186	779
Jelly Tip	each	152	634
Joy Bar	each	162	677
Vanilla Slices	100g	211	881
Fruju			
Grapefruit & Lemon	each	65	275
Orange Rush	each	73	306
Passionfruit & Orange Sorbet	each	65	275

DESSERTS

	QUANTITY	CALS	KJ
Pineapple Crush	each	72	302
Memphis Meltdown			
Big Bikkie	each	323	1350
Big Choc Brownie	each	311	1300
Big Hokey	each	349	1460
Gooey Caramel	each	361	1510
Gooey Raspberry	each	349	1460
Popsicle			
Blasts	each	77	322
Chocolate Milkshake Swirls	each	75	317
Lemonade	each	52	219
Slushy	each	139	578
Strawberry Milkshake Swirls	each	70	269
Tongue Twista	each	81	339
Traffic Light	each	54	225
Tropical Fruity	each	65	271
Trumpet			
Boysenberry	each	244	1020
Jelly Tip	each	245	1020
Strawberry	each	228	955
Triple Chocolate	each	252	1050
Vanilla	each	233	975
Tubs			
Blueberry Yoghurt	100g	150	633
Boysenberry Ripple	100g	203	847
Candy Floss	100g	206	859
Chocolate	100g	204	855
Cookies & Cream	100g	231	969
French Vanilla	100g	206	863
Go Go Banana	100g	207	866
Goody Goody Gum Drops	100g	226	945
Hokey Pokey	100g	221	926
Jelly Tip	100g	207	865
Light Hokey Pokey	100g	176	737
Light Vanilla	100g	162	678

	QUANTITY	CALS	KJ
Neopolitan	100g	221	926
Orange Choc Chip	100g	220	922
Passionfruit Yoghurt	100g	160	669
Raspberry Lemonade Fizz	100g	203	849
Strawberries & Cream	100g	207	866
Strawberry Yoghurt	100g	156	653
Swirly Caramel	100g	219	916
Vanilla	100g	206	863
WATTIE'S			
Creamed Rice			
Banana	100g	94	395
Chocolate 99% Fat Free	100g	102	430
Vanilla	100g	109	460
Vanilla 99% Fat Free	100g	100	420
WEIGHT WATCHERS			
Belgian Eclairs	100g	291	1220
Butterscotch Pudding	100g	272	720
Double Chocolate Pudding	100g	195	815
Ice Cream			
Berry Mudslide	100g	149	625
Creamy Vanilla	100g	137	575
Ice Cream Sundaes			
Double Chocolate	100g	188	790
Toffee Peach	100g	179	750
Jelly, all flavours	100mL	6	29
ZILCH			
Chocolate Ice Cream	100g	150	620
Passionfruit & Mango Frozen Yoghurt	100g	115	490
Vanilla Ice Cream	100g	150	620
Cones			
Wafer	each	118	494
Waffle	each	160	670
Toppings			
COTTEE'S, Choc Whizz, all flavours	100mL	633	2650
HERSHEY'S			

DESSERTS/DRESSINGS

	QUANTITY	CALS	KJ
Hot Fudge Topping	2 tbsp	120	502
Shell Topping	2 tbsp	100	418
HOMEBRAND			
Caramel	100mL	219	920
Chocolate	100mL	246	1030
Strawberry	100mL	241	1010
JOK'N'AL			
Boysenberry & Orange	2 tbsp	15	63
Passionfruit	2 tbsp	12	54
Raspberry	2 tbsp	12	52
Spiced Apple	2 tbsp	16	70
SELECT			
Dessert Sauce			
Mango & Passionfruit	100mL	210	880
Mixed Berry	100mL	191	800
Flavoured Coating, all flavours	100mL	628	2630

Dressings

	QUANTITY	CALS	KJ
ALFA ONE			
Aioli	100mL	58	1500
Creamy Mayo	100mL	372	1560
Real Mayonnaise	100g	657	2750
BEST FOODS			
Light Mayonnaise	1 tbsp	35	146
Real Mayonnaise	1 tbsp	90	376
BUDGET, Salad Dressing	100g	202	846
COTTERILL & ROUSE			
Balsamic	25g	28	118
Mango & Chilli	25g	25	106
Morroccan	25g	28	121
Thai Coriander & Lime	25g	31	133
DUKE'S Mayonnaise	14g	100	418
EDMONDS			
100% Fat Free French	20mL	15	65

	QUANTITY	CALS	KJ
100% Fat Free Italian	20mL	8	35
Balsamic	20mL	40	170
Caesar	20mL	64	270
Coleslaw	20mL	86	360
Light Whole Egg Mayonnaise	20g	64	270
Ranch	20mL	67	280
Thousand Island	20mL	57	240
Whole Egg Mayonnaise	20g	146	615
ETA			
Balsamic Vinaigrette	100mL	62	260
Caramelised Onion	100mL	163	685
Coleslaw	100mL	308	1290
Creamy			
Avocado & Garlic	100mL	353	1480
Caesar	100mL	442	1850
Garlic Mayonnaise	100mL	363	1520
Honey Mustard	100mL	363	1520
Potato Salad	100mL	358	1500
Ranch	100mL	308	1290
Southwest Chipotle	100mL	425	1780
Thousand Island	100mL	346	1450
Yoghurt & Garlic	100mL	289	1210
Lite & Free			
Balsamic Vinegar	100mL	71	300
Feta & Garlic	100mL	108	455
French	100mL	65	275
Honey Mustard	100mL	164	690
Italian	100mL	65	275
Lime & Coriander	100mL	75	315
Mayonnaise	100mL	161	675
Potato Salad	100mL	154	465
Salad Dressing	100mL	138	580
Mayonnaise	100mL	353	1480
Seafood Dressing	100mL	248	1470
Tartare	100mL	351	1470

DRESSINGS

	QUANTITY	CALS	KJ
HEINZ			
Dressing			
Balsamic	100mL	286	1200
French	100mL	344	1440
NZ Honey & 3 Mustard	100mL	501	2100
Parmesan Caesar	100mL	556	2330
Ranch	100mL	537	2250
Seriously Good			
Aioli	100mL	619	2590
Aioli, Lite	100mL	325	1360
Mayonnaise	100mL	650	2720
Mayonnaise, Lite	100mL	353	1480
Peri Peri Mayonnaise	100mL	614	2570
Tartare	100mL	571	2390
HOMEBRAND			
French	100mL	80	336
Italian	100mL	86	359
Mayonnaise 99% Fat Free	100mL	151	635
Potato Salad Dressing	100mL	207	867
KATO, Aioli	100g	614	2570
KRISPKUT			
Balsamic & Olive Oil Vinaigrette	50g	98	413
Blue Cheese	50g	227	952
Classic Caesar	50g	212	890
Creamy Ranch	50g	227	950
French Red Wine Vinaigrette	50g	120	501
Gourmet Hempseed & Honey	50g	112	472
Gourmet Japanese Style Sesame	50g	213	895
Gourmet Japanese Style Vinaigrette	50g	209	877
Italian Style White Wine Vinaigrette	50g	119	501
Mango Citrus Vinaigrette	50g	73	307
PAMS			
Avocado & Garlic Dressing	100mL	253	1060
Balsamic Vinaigrette	100mL	221	925
Classic Mayonnaise, American Style	100mL	738	3090

	QUANTITY	CALS	KJ
Coleslaw Dressing	100g	173	728
Hollandaise	100g	454	1900
Honey Mustard Dressing	100mL	291	1220
Lite Mayonnaise, American Style	100mL	348	1460
Lite Mayonnaise, Guilt Free	100g	95	400
Lite Dressing			
Balsamic	100mL	80	336
French	100mL	64	270
Honey & Mustard	100mL	123	515
Italian	100mL	65	272
Mayonnaise, Rich & Creamy	100mL	368	1540
Potato Salad Dressing	100g	216	905
Salad Dressing	100g	301	1260
Tartare Sauce	100g	432	1810
Thousand Island	100g	210	879
PAUL NEWMAN'S OWN			
Balsamic Vinaigrette	20mL	68	285
Caesar	20mL	93	390
Classic	20mL	76	320
Creamy Caesar	20mL	108	455
Light Balsamic Vinaigrette	20mL	31	130
Light Honey Mustard	20mL	46	195
Ranch	20mL	118	495
SELECT, Seafood Sauce	100mL	406	1700
WEIGHT WATCHERS			
Balsamic	100mL	72	305
Honey & Mustard	100mL	187	785

Drinks

Alcoholic Drinks			
BEER			
Black Ale	355mL	179	749
Dark	355mL	142	594
Draught	355mL	139	582

DRINKS

	QUANTITY	CALS	KJ
Guinness	355mL	176	736
Lager	355mL	153	640
Light	355mL	103	429
Low Alcohol	355mL	76	317
Stout	355mL	185	773
COCKTAILS			
Bloody Mary	114mL	48	201
Cosmopolitan	114mL	206	860
Daiquiri	114mL	216	904
Mai Tai	114mL	260	1087
Margarita	114mL	179	748
Martini			
Dry	114mL	206	860
Sweet	114mL	154	645
Piña Colada	133mL	245	1026
LIQUEUR			
Advocaat	30mL	85	355
Baileys Irish Cream	30mL	98	410
Bénédictine	30mL	90	376
Chartreuse	30mL	100	418
Crème de Cacao	30mL	100	418
Crème de Menthe	30mL	111	466
Curaçao	30mL	125	521
Galliano	30mL	100	418
Kirsch	30mL	80	334
Pernod	30mL	75	314
Schnapps	30mL	132	552
Tia Maria	30mL	90	376
Triple Sec	30mL	73	305
SPIRITS			
Bacardi	30mL	66	275
Brandy	30mL	65	274
Dubonnet	30mL	40	167
Gin	30mL	65	272
Madeira	30mL	47	197

	QUANTITY	CALS	KJ
Ouzo	30mL	103	431
Pimm's	30mL	48	200
Rum	30mL	65	272
Tequila	30mL	65	272
Vodka	30mL	73	304
Whisky	30mL	74	308
WINE			
Champagne	121mL	78	325
Chianti	121mL	100	419
Cider			
Dry	114mL	43	182
Sweet	114mL	64	268
Claret	150mL	123	516
Moselle	120mL	113	472
Port	60mL	94	394
Red, Cabernet	120mL	103	431
Reisling	120mL	97	406
Rosé	120mL	82	341
Sauterne	120mL	113	472
Sherry			
Cream	120mL	181	758
Dry	120mL	179	750
Sweet	120mL	181	758
White			
Dry	120mL	96	400
Medium	120mL	113	472
Cordial			
BAKER HALL CORDIALS			
Blackcurrant	100mL	32	133
Cranberry & Blackcurrant	100mL	35	145
Lemon & Barley	100mL	37	156
Lemon & Barley, Low Calorie	100mL	5	22
Lime Juice	100mL	23	97
Orange & Barley	100mL	37	153
Orange & Barley, Low Calorie	100mL	6	26

DRINKS

	QUANTITY	CALS	KJ
BARKER'S			
Apricot Blush	100mL	33	141
Berrylife	100mL	34	144
Blackcurrant	100mL	40	162
Blackcurrant with Boysenberry	100mL	40	170
Blackcurrant with Cranberry	100mL	40	169
Blackcurrant with Raspberry	100mL	40	185
Lemon & Barley	100mL	34	146
Lemon & Honey	100mL	29	123
Lemon & Lime	100mL	35	148
Lemon, Honey & Ginger	100mL	40	171
Lime Juice	100mL	30	127
Limes with Elderflower	100mL	30	127
Lite Blackcurrant	100mL	19	79
Lite Lemon & Barley	100mL	19	80
Orange & Barley with Passionfruit	100mL	34	145
Unsweetened Blackcurrant	100mL	14	62
Vegelife	100mL	42	179
BUDERIM			
Diet Lemon, Lime & Bitters	100mL	14	62
Ginger Refresher	100mL	59	230
Ginger Revitalise	100mL	16	69
Lemon, Lime & Bitters	100mL	44	185
PAMS			
Blackcurrant	100mL	31	133
Lemon & Barley	100mL	34	146
Lime	100mL	43	84
Orange & Barley	100mL	34	144
RIBENA, Blackcurrant	100mL	50	210
ROBINSONS			
Apple & Blackcurrant	100mL	7	30
Orange	100mL	9	38
ROSE'S			
Lemon	100mL	37	156
Lime	100mL	26	112

	QUANTITY	CALS	KJ
SCHWEPPES			
Lemon Squash	100mL	30	126
Lime	100mL	30	128
Raspberry	100mL	31	133
SIGNATURE RANGE			
Lemon & Barley	100mL	41	175
Lime	100mL	28	118
Orange & Barley	100mL	39	166
THRIFTEE			
Blackcurrant	100mL	1	2
Lime	100mL	1	2
Orange Mango	100mL	1	2
Pineapple Orange	100mL	1	2
Raspberry	100mL	1	2
Energy Drinks			
DEMON	100mL	52	218
LIFT PLUS, Original	250mL	125	526
LOADED			
Isotonic, Desert Storm	100mL	31	132
Zero, Avalanche Blast	100mL	1	5
MONSTER	100mL	46	194
MOTHER			
Black	100mL	47	195
Inferno	100mL	47	196
NOS, Original	100mL	42	175
PHOENIX, Pomegranate	100mL	44	185
RED BULL			
Original	100mL	45	192
Sugarfree	100mL	3	14
V			
Blue	100mL	59	247
Graphite	100mL	58	243
Original	100mL	46	195
Sugarfree	100mL	30	127

DRINKS

	QUANTITY	CALS	KJ
Hot Drinks (prepared as directed, unless stated otherwise)			
Coffee, café style			
Black	1 cup	5	21
Cappuccino, Standard Milk	1 cup	165	690
Cappuccino, Trim Milk	1 cup	96	402
Flat White, Standard Milk	1 cup	168	705
Flat White, Trim Milk	1 cup	93	390
Latte, Standard Milk	1 cup	168	705
Latte, Trim Milk	1 cup	97	405
Mochaccino, Standard Milk	1 cup	214	894
Mochaccino, Trim Milk	1 cup	150	627
AVALANCHE			
Cafe			
Cappuccino	100mL	43	181
Flat White	100mL	34	45
Mochaccino	100mL	41	174
Divine Drinking Chocolate	100mL	58	246
Marshmallow Melt Drinking Chocolate	100mL	58	246
CADBURY			
Drinking Chocolate	15g	156	653
Drinking Chocolate, Caramel	15g	156	654
Drinking Chocolate, Mint	15g	156	653
GREGG'S			
Café Gold Coffee Mix			
Cappuccino	100mL	48	199
Caramel Latte	100mL	49	206
Flat White	100mL	40	168
Hazelnut Latte	100mL	50	210
Hot Chocolate	100mL	53	222
Mint Choc Latte	100mL	50	211
Mochaccino	100mL	54	226
Spicy Chai Latte	100mL	233	977
HORLICKS	per serve	233	977

	QUANTITY	CALS	KJ
JARRAH			
Bavarian Bliss	100mL	34	143
Brazil Delight	100mL	32	135
Cheeky 'Cino	100mL	38	156
French Liaison	100mL	34	143
Latte, Vanilla Thriller	100mL	38	159
Swiss Moments	100mL	31	131
Vienna Velvet	100mL	33	136
White Choc-a-Mocha	100mL	36	152
MOCCONA			
Coffee Mix			
Cappuccino	100mL	39	163
Cappuccino Strong	100mL	38	160
Caramel Latte	100mL	40	167
Latte	100mL	44	185
Mochaccino	100mL	37	153
NESCAFÉ			
Azera			
Cappuccino	100mL	39	160
Latte	100mL	42	175
Café Menu			
Cappuccino, Decaf	100mL	41	170
Cappuccino, Normal	100mL	39	165
Cappuccino, Skim	100mL	29	125
Cappuccino, Strong	100mL	38	160
Caramel Latte	100mL	48	205
Flat White	100mL	64	270
Hazelnut Latte	100mL	53	225
Mocha	100mL	50	210
Mocha, Skim	100mL	38	160
Vanilla Latte	100mL	53	225
NESTLÉ			
MILO	per serve	141	590
NESQUIK			
Banana	per serve	149	625

DRINKS

	QUANTITY	CALS	KJ
Chocolate	per serve	150	630
Strawberry	per serve	150	630
Ovaltine	per serve	200	835
PAMS			
Cappuccino	100mL	39	166
Mochaccino	100mL	47	197
PHOENIX			
Chai	100mL	76	319
Lemon Toddy	100mL	32	138
SELECT			
Cappuccino	100g	37	154
Mochaccino	100g	53	220
WEIGHT WATCHERS, Drinking Chocolate	per serve	117	490
Instant Drinks			
MOLLOYS, all flavours	100mL	20	83
PAMS			
Apple & Berry	100mL	27	116
Lemon & Barley	100mL	27	116
Lemon & Lime	100mL	27	116
Naval Orange	100mL	27	116
Orange & Mango	100mL	27	117
Passionfruit & Orange	100mL	27	115
Pineapple	100mL	27	116
Raspberry	100mL	27	117
Tropical Orange	100mL	27	117
RARO			
Guava Mango Pineapple	100mL	32	132
Guava Orange	100mL	32	131
Lemonade	100mL	32	132
Mango Orange	100mL	32	132
Passionfruit Orange	100mL	32	132
Passionfruit Pineapple	100mL	32	132
Pineapple	100mL	32	133
Pineapple Orange	100mL	32	132
Raspberry	100mL	32	131

	QUANTITY	CALS	KJ
Strawberry Passionfruit	100mL	32	132
Sweet Mandarin	100mL	32	132
Sweet Naval Orange	100mL	32	132
Tropical	100mL	32	132
REFRESH			
Apple Berry	100mL	31	131
Breakfast Orange	100mL	31	132
Mango Orange	100mL	31	129
Passionfruit Orange	100mL	31	130
Peacharine	100mL	31	131
Pear Berry	100mL	31	131
Pineapple Orange	100mL	31	131
Sweet Florida Orange	100mL	31	129
Sweet Naval Orange	100mL	31	131
VITAFRESH			
Blackcurrant	100mL	27	112
Crisp Apple	100mL	27	112
Hawaiian Pineapple	100mL	26	111
Jamaican Lime	100mL	27	111
Orange & Mango	100mL	26	110
Raspberry	100mL	27	112
Sweet Naval Orange	100mL	26	111
Tutti Frutti Blue	100mL	26	111
White Peach & Passionfruit	100mL	26	111
WEIGHT WATCHERS, Sweet Naval Orange	100mL	14	20
Juices			
ARANO			
Classic Range			
100% NZ Orange	100mL	50	210
Apricot with Apple	100mL	43	184
Grapefruit	100mL	30	128
Peach with Apple	100mL	46	196
Pear with Apple	100mL	47	200
Plum with Apple	100mL	43	184

DRINKS

	QUANTITY	CALS	KJ
Smoothies			
Berry	100mL	67	283
Feijoa	100mL	61	259
Spirulina	100mL	53	224
Vanilla Bean & Honey	100mL	81	340
White Label			
Gisborne Tangelo	100mL	50	212
Gisborne Valencia	100mL	55	233
Kerikeri Valencia	100mL	55	233
CERES			
Guava	240mL	120	502
Litchi	240mL	120	502
Mango	240mL	120	502
Medley of Fruits	240mL	130	543
CHARLIE'S			
Honest Juices			
Apple	100mL	45	191
Orange	100mL	38	162
Honest Juice Drinks			
Apple	100mL	23	95
Orange	100mL	22	91
Honest Whole Fruit Smoothies			
Berry	100mL	56	235
Feijoa	100mL	55	232
Guava	100mL	54	226
Mango	100mL	54	226
Spirulina	100mL	68	288
Juice 50% Less Sugar			
Blackcurrant & Apple	100mL	33	140
Orange	100mL	32	135
Raspberry & Apple	100mL	33	140
Summer Fruits	100mL	33	140
Quenchers			
Blackcurrant	100mL	45	191
Feijoa	100mL	45	192

	QUANTITY	CALS	KJ
Lemonade	100mL	45	190
Limeade	100mL	44	188
Mango Orange	100mL	45	190
Raspberry	100mL	46	193
Sicilian Blood Orange	100mL	45	192
White Peach & Passionfruit	100mL	45	192
FRESH UP			
Apple & Nectarine	100mL	44	187
Apple & Orange	100mL	43	181
Apple & Pineapple	100mL	39	165
Apple & Summ...Ahh... Fruits	100mL	43	180
Crisp Apple	100mL	44	187
Harvest Red Apple	100mL	40	170
GOLDEN CIRCLE			
Golden Pash	100mL	47	200
Nectar			
Apricot	100mL	64	270
Guava	100mL	50	210
Mango	100mL	50	210
Pineapple	100mL	51	215
Pineapple & Mango	100mL	69	190
Tropical Punch	100mL	47	200
GREENWAYS			
100% Pure Grape	100mL	69	290
Apple	100mL	45	192
Apple & Grape	100mL	52	221
H2COCO			
Pineapple	100mL	21	90
Pomegranate & Acai	100mL	21	89
Pure	100mL	21	90
JUST JUICE			
50% Less Sugar			
Orange	100mL	23	97
Pear & Apple	100mL	27	116
Tropical	100mL	31	131

DRINKS

	QUANTITY	CALS	KJ
Orange	100mL	45	191
Orange & Apple	100mL	46	196
Orange & Mango	100mL	49	206
Pear & Apple	100mL	47	200
Pineapple & Guava	100mL	52	221
Strawberry & Kiwifruit	100mL	46	193
Tropical	100mL	49	208
KERI			
Fruit Drink			
5 Fruits	100mL	48	205
Apple	100mL	45	187
Apple, Orange & Mango	100mL	46	195
Blackcurrant	100mL	42	178
Cranberry	100mL	51	217
Cranberry Lite	100mL	6	26
Kids Apple & Blackcurrant	100mL	37	156
Kids Tropical Burst	100mL	37	157
Orange	100mL	51	215
Orange with Apple Base	100mL	42	179
Pineapple & Passionfruit	100mL	47	198
Pulpy Orange	100mL	43	175
Pulpy Tropical	100mL	44	188
Tropical	100mL	44	186
Premium			
Cranberry & Grapefruit	100mL	52	218
Grapefruit	100mL	39	164
Orange	100mL	42	178
Pineapple	100mL	44	186
Spicy Tomato	100mL	28	119
LANGERS			
Cranberry	100mL	140	585
Diet Cranberry	100mL	30	125
MCCOY			
Cranberry	100mL	49	207
Dark Grape	100mL	58	245

	QUANTITY	CALS	KJ
Grapefruit	100mL	37	155
Orange	100mL	42	178
Pineapple	100mL	42	177
Ruby Red Grapefruit	100mL	50	210
Tomato	100mL	23	100
NEKTA			
Kiwi	100mL	44	187
Kiwi & Aloe Vera	100mL	44	187
NUJU, Pure Coconut Water	100mL	17	71
OCEAN SPRAY			
Cranberry Blackcurrant	100mL	53	221
Cranberry Classic	100mL	46	192
Cranberry Light	100mL	8	33
Cranberry Pomegranate	100mL	48	200
Raspberry & Cranberry	100mL	48	201
Refreshers Cranberry	100mL	48	201
Refreshers Light Cranberry	100mL	8	33
Ruby Red & Grapefruit	100mL	50	209
PAMS			
Original Orange	100mL	48	201
Tropical with Apple Base	100mL	43	181
PHOENIX			
Apple	100mL	47	198
Apple & Pomegranate	100mL	47	199
Apple, Peach & Raspberry	100mL	47	199
Blackcurrant & Apple	100mL	47	199
Feijoa & Apple	100mL	47	198
Guava & Apple	100mL	47	198
Mango Passion & Apple	100mL	47	199
Orange Mango & Apple	100mL	47	199
Pear & Apple	100mL	45	191
Sparkling Blackcurrant	100mL	29	122
Sparkling Blood Orange	100mL	41	175
Sparkling Cranberry & Lime	100mL	36	152
Sparkling Feijoa	100mL	35	150

DRINKS

	QUANTITY	CALS	KJ
Sparking Juicy Apple	100mL	46	193
REJUVA, Aloe Vera	100mL	44	186
RIBENA			
Blackcurrant	100mL	42	177
Blackcurrant & Cranberry	100mL	41	173
SELECT			
Cranberry Fruit Drink	100mL	47	199
Real Juice, Multipack			
Apple	100mL	47	197
Orange	100mL	41	174
Tropical	100mL	48	204
SIGNATURE RANGE			
Apple	100mL	40	168
Orange	100mL	44	186
Orange & Mango	100mL	42	179
Tropical	100mL	40	171
SIMPLY SQUEEZED			
Berry-Fruit Smoothie	350mL	235	987
Feijoa Smoothie	350mL	226	949
Fruit Smoothie with Spirulina	350mL	182	764
Orange	350mL	148	623
SUNRAYSIA			
Apple	100mL	43	181
Apple & Elderflower	100mL	36	152
Apple & Raspberry	100mL	42	175
Carrot, Orange & Apple	100mL	45	186
Cranberry	100mL	79	328
Heart Beet	100mL	79	328
Mixed Vegetable & Apple	100mL	42	175
Orange	100mL	48	201
Pomegranate	100mL	48	201
Prune	100mL	77	308
Red Grape, Raspberry & Acai	100mL	70	294
SUNSWEET, Prune Juice	100mL	19	82

	QUANTITY	CALS	KJ
THEXTONS			
Blackcurrant	100mL	48	203
Cranberry	100mL	50	211
Orange	100mL	37	156
Orange & Mango	100mL	37	158
Orange & Peach	100mL	39	166
V8			
Citrus Fusion	100mL	49	187
Orange Mango Passion	100mL	47	199
Tropical Fusion	100mL	43	181
Vegetable Juice			
Breakfast & Fibre	100mL	47	197
Low Sodium	100mL	21	89
Original	100mL	21	90
Soft Drinks			
APPLEMAID, Sparkling Apple Juice	100mL	48	200
APPLETISER			
Appletiser	100mL	43	182
Grapetiser, Red	100mL	52	218
Grapetiser, White	100mL	54	227
BUNDABERG			
Blood Orange	100mL	49	207
Creaming Soda	100mL	45	189
Diet Ginger Beer	100mL	8	34
Diet Lemon, Lime & Bitters	100mL	8	34
Diet Sarsaparilla	100mL	8	34
Ginger Beer	100mL	43	184
Guava	100mL	46	196
Lemon, Lime & Bitters	100mL	48	201
Lime	100mL	46	196
Peachee	100mL	46	196
Passionfruit	100mL	49	206
Pink Grapefruit	100mL	45	192
Sarsaparilla	100mL	50	211

DRINKS

	QUANTITY	CALS	KJ
CH'I			
Original	100mL	40	167
Zero	100mL	1	5
COCA-COLA			
Coca-Cola	100mL	43	180
Coca-Cola Vanilla	100mL	44	185
Coca-Cola Zero	100mL	0	1
Coca-Cola Zero Vanilla	100mL	0	1
Diet Coca-Cola	100mL	0	1
Diet Coca-Cola, Caffeine Free	100mL	0	1
Diet L&P	100mL	1	5
Diet Lift	100mL	1	8
Fanta	100mL	50	212
Fanta Grape	100mL	155	234
Fanta Raspberry	100mL	48	205
L&P	100mL	44	186
Lift	100mL	45	192
Sprite	100mL	41	172
Sprite Zero	100mL	1	4
Vanilla Coke	100mL	44	185
DR PEPPER	240mL	100	478
FRANK			
Sparkling Soda & Key Lime	100mL	21	90
Sparkling Tangy Blood Orange	100mL	43	180
Sparkling Zesty Lemonade	100mL	45	190
HOMEBRAND			
Cola	100mL	31	130
Diet Lemonade	100mL	0	4
Ginger Beer	100mL	32	136
Lemon Crush	100mL	33	140
Lemonade	100mL	28	120
Lime	100mL	31	130
Orange	100mL	35	150
Pineapple	100mL	31	130
Raspberry	100mL	33	140

	QUANTITY	CALS	KJ
Soda Water	100mL	0	0
JUST JUICE BUBBLES			
Lemon Crush	100mL	42	176
Lite Tropical	100mL	20	87
Orange & Mango	100mL	43	182
Tropical	100mL	42	177
LOL			
BCurrent	100mL	47	200
Razz Bri	100mL	47	200
Tropkl	100mL	48	205
MAC'S			
Feijoa & Pear	100mL	32	135
Ginger Beer	100mL	35	148
Green Apple	100mL	33	140
Lemon Crush	100mL	32	137
PAMS			
Classic Soda Water	100mL	1	5
Cola	100mL	31	132
Creaming Soda	100mL	31	131
Diet Cola	100mL	3	6
Diet Ginger Beer	100mL	0	4
Diet Indian Tonic Water	100mL	1	5
Diet Lemonade	100mL	1	5
Dry Ginger Ale	100mL	28	120
Ginger Beer	100mL	40	170
Grape	100mL	49	207
Green Apple	100mL	36	151
Ice Cream Soda	100mL	34	146
Indian Tonic Water	100mL	26	112
Lemon	100mL	33	139
Lemon, Lime & Bitters	100mL	29	124
Lemonade	100mL	33	142
Lime	100mL	36	151
Orange	100mL	34	144
Passionfruit	100mL	30	129

DRINKS

	QUANTITY	CALS	KJ
Pineapple	100mL	34	146
Raspberry	100mL	32	137
Soda, Twist of Lemon	100mL	21	92
Sparkling Red Grape Juice	100mL	79	333
Sparkling White Grape Juice	100mL	79	333
Tropical	100mL	40	169
PEPSICO			
7UP	100mL	43	181
7UP Light	100mL	1	5
Mountain Dew	100mL	47	199
Pepsi	100mL	41	175
Pepsi Max	100mL	0	1
PHOENIX ORGANICS			
Cola	100mL	45	188
Ginger Beer	100mL	36	153
Honey Cola	100mL	44	188
Lemon, Lime & Bitters	100mL	40	168
Lemonade	100mL	45	150
Light Cola	100mL	26	110
Orange Fizz	100mL	35	207
Raspberry Fizz	100mL	49	207
Royal Crown Cola	100mL	50	213
SAXBYS			
Diet Ginger Beer	100mL	0	2
Ginger Beer	100mL	53	223
Ginger, Lime & Bitters	100mL	45	189
Ginger Twist	100mL	41	172
SCHWEPPES			
Classic Diet Lemonade	100mL	1	4
Diet Dry Ginger Ale	100mL	1	5
Diet Tonic	100mL	1	7
Dry Ginger Ale	100mL	40	171
Dry Lemonade	100mL	44	185
Ginger Beer	100mL	47	197
Ginger Beer, Light	100mL	1	4

	QUANTITY	CALS	KJ
Lemon, Lime & Bitters	100mL	44	186
Lime Cordial	100mL	37	158
Raspberry Cordial	100mL	41	173
Soda	100mL	0	0
Soda with a Twist	100mL	21	90
Sparkling Diet Lemonade	100mL	1	4
Sparkling Duet	100mL	54	229
Sparkling Ice Cream Soda	100mL	53	224
Sparkling Lemon	100mL	41	175
Sparkling Lemonade	100mL	42	177
Sparkling Lime	100mL	48	203
Sparkling Raspberry	100mL	48	205
Tonic	100mL	37	156
Traditional Lemonade	100mL	43	183
SELECT			
Apple & Blackcurrant	100mL	42	178
Fruit Fizz	100mL	37	158
Lemon	100mL	50	210
Lemonade	100mL	47	200
Orange	100mL	46	193
Raspberry	100mL	41	174
Tropical	100mL	50	210
SIGNATURE RANGE			
Cola	100mL	38	160
Dry Ginger Ale	100mL	43	182
Diet Lemon, Lime & Bitters	100mL	0	4
Diet Lemonade	100mL	0	2
Diet Tonic Water	100mL	0	4
Dry Lemonade	100mL	43	182
Ginger Beer	100mL	44	187
Lemon	100mL	60	250
Lemon, Lime & Bitters	100mL	33	140
Lemonade	100mL	40	170
Orange	100mL	50	210
Soda Water	100mL	0	0

DRINKS

	QUANTITY	CALS	KJ
Tonic Water	100mL	33	140
SOUL VIRGIN, Mojito	100mL	40	170
360			
Ginger Beer	100mL	32	134
Lemonade	100mL	37	134
Tidal Wave	100mL	32	134
Sports Drinks			
E2			
Apple	100mL	39	167
Blackcurrant	100mL	41	174
Lemon Lime	100mL	39	165
Mango, Passion & Apple	100mL	39	166
Orange	100mL	39	165
GATORADE, all flavours	100mL	24	103
GFORCE			
Apple Blackcurrant	100mL	43	184
Mango Pineapple	100mL	45	191
Orange Mandarin	100mL	42	177
LUCOZADE SPORT	100mL	28	117
MIZONE			
Crisp Apple	100mL	11	49
Lime	100mL	11	49
Mandarin	100mL	11	49
Peach	100mL	11	50
POWERADE			
Berry Ice	100mL	31	131
Charge Down	100mL	31	129
Lemon Lime	100mL	31	131
Mountain Blast	100mL	32	133
VITASPORT, Water Booster			
Lemon Lime	100mL	1	5
Mixed Berry	100mL	1	4
Orange Mango	100mL	1	4

	QUANTITY	CALS	KJ
Water, Flavoured			
H2GO			
Boysenberry	100mL	1	8
Lime	100mL	2	9
Summer Fruits	100mL	1	8

Eggs

	QUANTITY	CALS	KJ
Boiled	1 large	78	326
Fried in Vegetable Oil	1 large	119	497
Poached	1 large	84	350
Raw			
White	1 large	16	67
Yolk	1 large	54	226
Scrambled with Milk	1 large	80	334

Ethnic Meals

CHINESE	QUANTITY	CALS	KJ
Barbecue Spare Ribs	100g	118	493
Beef, Black Bean	100g	77	323
Chicken & Cashew Nuts	100g	111	466
Chicken & Sweet Corn Soup	100g	57	238
Chicken Chop Suey	100g	104	435
Chow Mein	100g	145	605
Dim Sim	each	100	419
Egg Fu Yung	100g	185	773
Egg Noodles, _cooked_	1 cup	221	926
Fried Rice	100g	157	651
Lemon Chicken	1 cup	500	2095
Lychees	each	6	25
Pork Chop Suey	100g	123	513
Pork with Garlic & Chilli	100g	183	766
Prawn Chop Suey	350g	215	900
Prawn Crackers	10 crackers	100	419

ETHNIC MEALS

	QUANTITY	CALS	KJ
Spring Roll	each	319	1330
Sweet & Sour			
Fish	100g	139	579
Pork	100g	238	992
Vegetables, *stir fried*	100g	118	494
Wonton Soup	220g	178	745
INDIAN			
Aloo Samosa (potato filling)	each	200	838
Beef Madras	100g	203	848
Butter Chicken	100g	191	800
Chapati	100g	298	1248
Chicken Masala	100g	191	800
Chicken Pilaf	1 cup	220	921
Dhal Makhani	100g	163	678
Korma, Beef	100g	219	915
Mulligatawny Soup	1 cup	230	963
Poppadam, *fried*	30g	120	502
Pork Vindaloo Curry	per serve	620	2597
Rogan Josh, Lamb	100g	135	564
Roti	each	60	251
Saag Gosht (lamb, spinach)	1 cup	573	2400
Tandoori Chicken			
Breast	per serve	260	1089
Leg or Thigh	per serve	300	1257
JAPANESE			
Inari-zushi (bean curd pouches with sushi)	each	130	544
Miso Soup with Tofu Pieces	1 cup	66	276
Nigiri Sushi (fish wrapped)	2 rolls	73	301
Nori Maki-zushi (seaweed wrapped)	each	70	293
Sake Rice Wine	30mL	39	163
Sashimi (raw fish)			
Kingfish	30g	30	125
Mackerel	30g	60	251
Salmon	30g	60	251

	QUANTITY	CALS	KJ
Sea Bass	30g	30	125
Tuna	30g	40	167
Sukiyaki Beef, Tofu & Vegetables	250g	362	1516
Tempura Prawns & Vegetables	5 pieces	350	1466
Teppan-Yaki Steak	280g	470	1969
Teriyaki Beef	110g	350	1466
MEXICAN			
Bean Burrito	each	350	1466
Beef Burrito	each	280	1173
Enchilada	each	300	1257
Nachos (cheese, beans & ground beef)	255g	569	2390
Taco (meat, cheese, salad)	100g	221	920
Tortilla/Tostados with Beef	100g	190	796
MIDDLE EASTERN			
Cabbage Roll	each	223	934
Calamari (squid)	170g	350	1466
Couscous	1 cup	176	737
Kebab, Lamb	each	210	879
Kibbi	each	274	1148
Moussaka	350g	509	2132
Souvlaki	each	365	1529
Tabbouleh (cracked wheat salad)	1 cup	94	393
Taramasalata (fish roe)	1 tbsp	80	335
Vine Leaves, *stuffed*	2 small rolls	200	838
THAI			
Curry			
Green, with Chicken	1 cup	557	2340
Green, with Pork	1 cup	476	1994
Massaman	1 cup	676	2832
Red, with Beef	1 cup	449	1881
Fish Cake, *fried*	100g	238	991
Pad Thai	100g	199	825
Penang, Beef	250g	534	2237
Prawns, Garlic	3 pieces	84	349

ETHNIC MEALS/FAST FOOD

	QUANTITY	CALS	KJ
Salad, Beef	100g	94	390
Satay, Pork	172g	411	1722
Tom Yum Soup, Chicken	100g	40	167

Fast Food

BURGER KING

Breakfast

Bacon & Egg Muffin	each	318	1334
BLT Wrap	each	391	1639
Brekkie Wrap	each	591	2476
Egg Muffin	each	264	1108
Hash Bites	each	237	995
Hotcakes	each	430	1803
King Muffin	each	666	2789
King's Brekkie	each	698	2921
Muffin & Jam	each	244	1021
Sausage & Egg Muffin	each	417	1745
Yoghurt Berry Pottle	each	429	1796

Burgers

Bacon Double Cheeseburger	each	496	2078
Bacon Relish TenderCrisp	each	761	3186
BBQ Beef Burger	each	338	1415
BBQ Rodeo	each	435	1821
BK Chicken	each	669	2802
BK Chicken, Hawaiian	each	831	3478
BLT Steakhouse	each	814	3406
Brewers' Steakhouse	each	798	3343
Cheeseburger	each	312	1306
Creamy Mayo Cheeseburger	each	379	1587
Double Cheeseburger	each	456	1911
Grabba	each	336	1409
Hamburger	each	268	1124
Honey Mustard TenderCrisp	each	706	2958
Salad Burger	each	585	2449

	QUANTITY	CALS	KJ
Streaky Bacon Steakhouse	each	820	3431
TenderCrisp Original	each	692	2899
TenderCrisp Spicy	each	600	2514
Tender Grill, Flatbread	each	358	1520
The King's Fish Burger	each	473	1982
Triple Cheeseburger	each	607	2541
Whopper	each	633	2649
Whopper, Cheese	each	720	3013
Whopper, Double	each	861	3606
Whopper JR	each	338	1416
Whopper JR, Cheese	each	381	1598
Whopper JR, Lite Mayo	each	280	1174
Whopper, Lite Mayo	each	522	2187
Chicken Tenders, 3 pack	per serve	173	725
Desserts			
HERSHEY'S Chocolate Pie	each	426	1786
Soft Serve Cone	each	210	881
Sundae, Caramel	each	231	969
Sundae, Chocolate	each	231	969
Sundae, Plain	each	140	588
Sundae, Strawberry	each	199	833
Salads			
Side	each	16	68
TenderCrisp	each	261	1096
TenderGrill	each	167	701
Sides			
Beer Battered Onion Rings	per serve	246	1030
Fries, Regular	per serve	298	1248
Onion Rings	per serve	263	1101
Wraps			
Honey Mustard TenderCrisp	each	396	1658
Honey Mustard TenderGrill	each	301	1263
Sweet Chilli TenderCrisp	each	396	1660
Sweet Chilli TenderGrill	each	302	1265
Tomato Relish TenderCrisp	each	395	1656

	QUANTITY	CALS	KJ
Tomato Relish TenderGrill	each	301	1260
BURGER WISCONSIN			
Burgers, Grand			
Beef & Avo & Bacon	each	897	3757
Beef & Cheese	each	875	3663
Beef & Garlic	each	777	3251
Beef & Hot Chilli Tomato Salsa	each	777	3252
Beef, Mushrooms & Blue Cheese	each	807	3377
Big Island (breast)	each	960	4020
Big Island (tenderloins)	each	805	3369
Chicken, Avocado & Bacon (breast)	each	910	3809
Chicken, Avocado & Bacon (tenderloins)	each	760	3180
Chicken, Camembert & Cranberry (breast)	each	889	3721
Chicken, Camembert & Cranberry (tenderloins)	each	733	3070
Chicken, Chilli Jam & Cheese (breast)	each	922	3860
Chicken, Chilli Jam & Cheese (tenderloins)	each	767	3213
Chicken Satay (breast)	each	914	3828
Chicken Satay (tenderloins)	each	759	3177
Chicken Tandoori	each	740	3099
Fish, Coriander & Lime	each	751	3145
Gluten Free Chicken	each	569	2381
Kiwi Classic	each	1081	4245
Love Me Tender	each	690	2887
McCartney	each	862	3610
Minted Lamb	each	754	3158
Pestarella	each	966	4042
Rocket	each	1019	4266
The Full Monty	each	1246	5215
Vegetarian Deluxe	each	1029	4308
Venison & Otago Plum	each	790	3307
Junior			
Beef & Cheese Burger	per serve	619	2590
Chicken Burger	per serve	573	2399

	QUANTITY	CALS	KJ
Crumbed NZ Catch Fish Fillet & Fries	per serve	674	2823
Tempura Chicken Nibbles, 3 pack, & Fries	per serve	743	3110

Sides

	QUANTITY	CALS	KJ
Crispy Crumbed Onion Rings	per serve	449	1880
Kumara Fries	per serve	553	2317
Potato Fries	per serve	478	2002
Seasoned Wedges	per serve	545	2284
Tempura Chicken Nibbles	per serve	442	1851

CARL'S JNR

Breakfast

	QUANTITY	CALS	KJ
Bacon, Egg & Cheese Sandwich	each	227	498
Breakfast Burger	each	886	3710
Deluxe Platter	per serve	813	3397
Hash Rounds	per serve	436	1820
Monster Breakfast Sandwich	each	576	2410
Pancakes Platter	per serve	552	2310
Sausage, Egg & Cheese Sandwich	each	213	1614
Super Deluxe Platter	per serve	1050	4388

Burgers

	QUANTITY	CALS	KJ
Double Western Bacon Cheeseburger	each	947	3960
Famous Star with Cheese	each	663	2770
Guacamole Bacon Thickburger	each	1013	4240
Jalapeño Thickburger	each	903	3780
Kids Cheeseburger	each	441	1850
Kids Hamburger	each	392	3780
Low Carb Thickburger	each	594	2490
Original Thickburger	each	850	3550
Portobello Mushroom	each	687	2870
Portobello Mushroom Thickburger	each	872	3650
Super Star with Cheese	each	838	3500
The Big Carl	each	845	3540
Western Bacon Cheeseburger	each	789	3300
Western Bacon Thickburger	each	1247	5220

Chicken & Other Choices

FAST FOOD

	QUANTITY	CALS	KJ
Bacon Swiss Crispy Hand-Breaded Chicken Tender Sandwich	each	727	3040
Buttermilk Ranch Hand-Breaded Chicken Tender Sandwich	each	587	2460
Carl's Catch Fish Sandwich	each	1077	4510
Charbroiled BBQ Chicken Sandwich	each	267	1120
Charbroiled Chicken Club Sandwich	each	450	1880
Charbroiled Santa Fe Chicken Sandwich	each	495	2070
Hand-Breaded Chicken Tenders, 3 pieces	per serve	247	1030
Honey Mustard Hand-Breaded Chicken Tender Sandwich	each	563	2360
Kids Hand-Breaded Chicken Tenders, 2 pieces	per serve	161	680
Desserts			
Oreo Ice Cream Sandwich	per serve	237	990
Passionfruit Cheesecake	per serve	597	2500
Strawberry Cheesecake	per serve	602	2520
Salads, Without Dressings			
Charbroiled Chicken	each	136	570
Crispy Chicken	each	222	930
Side	each	125	520
Sides			
Chili Cheese Fries	per serve	781	3160
CrissCut Fries	per serve	451	1890
Fried Zucchini	per serve	330	1380
Natural-Cut Fries	per serve	434	1820
Onion Rings	per serve	535	2240
DOMINO'S PIZZA			
Breads & Chips			
Cheesy Garlic Bread	60g	179	750
Chips	350g	703	2940
Garlic Bread	28g	80	336
Wedges	300g	538	2250
Cheesy Crust Base			
Bacon & Mushroom	per slice	255	1070

	QUANTITY	CALS	KJ
Bangers & Beef	per slice	243	1020
Beef & Onion	per slice	250	1050
Ham & Cheese	per slice	237	922
Ham & Tomato	per slice	255	1070
Hawaiian	per slice	244	1020
Margherita	per slice	225	942
Pepperoni	per slice	224	938
Sausage Sensation	per slice	269	1130
Vege Trio	per slice	223	934
Chicken Sides			
Cayenne Chicken Wings	34g	74	309
Mild Kickers	25g	42	174
Spicy Kickers	25g	45	190
Classic Base			
Bacon & Mushroom	per slice	190	794
Bangers & Beef	per slice	202	844
BBQ Hawaiian	per slice	203	850
Beef & Onion	per slice	185	775
Cheese	per slice	174	726
Chicken & Camembert	per slice	198	830
Chicken & Cranberry	per slice	189	789
Deli Vege	per slice	158	660
Grand Supreme	per slice	236	987
Ham & Cheese	per slice	172	720
Ham & Tomato	per slice	191	798
Hawaiian	per slice	179	749
Loaded Meatlovers	per slice	222	929
Margherita	per slice	178	746
Pepperoni	per slice	183	765
Pepperoni & Parmesan	per slice	234	980
Sausage Sensation	per slice	220	920
Vege Trio	per slice	158	662
Deep Pan Base			
Bacon & Mushroom	per slice	233	977
Bangers & Beef	per slice	245	1030

FAST FOOD

	QUANTITY	CALS	KJ
Beef & Onion	per slice	229	957
Cheese	per slice	217	909
Ham & Cheese	per slice	216	903
Ham & Tomato	per slice	234	981
Hawaiian	per slice	223	931
Margherita	per slice	204	855
Pepperoni	per slice	223	935
Sausage Sensation	per slice	246	1030
Vege Trio	per slice	202	845
Desserts			
Battered Bananas	25g	59	245
Chocolate Brownies	15g	73	306
Chocolate Lava Cake	90g	374	1570
Chocolate Mousse	100g	385	1600
Dutch Pancakes	107g	441	1850
White Choc Panna Cotta	100g	336	1410
Gluten Free Base			
Apricot Chicken	per slice	151	633
Cheese	per slice	140	584
Garlic Prawn	per slice	146	612
Ham & Cheese	per slice	138	577
Hawaiian	per slice	144	604
Margherita	per slice	127	533
Pepperoni	per slice	153	638
Peri Peri Beef	per slice	183	764
Peri Peri Chicken	per slice	151	632
Peri Peri Vege	per slice	163	681
Trio of Veg	per slice	124	521
Vegorama	per slice	132	551
Thin Base			
Bacon & Mushroom	per slice	197	825
Bangers & Beef	per slice	206	863
Beef & Onion	per slice	195	818
Ham & Cheese	per slice	179	751
Ham & Tomato	per slice	195	817

	QUANTITY	CALS	KJ
Hawaiian	per slice	186	780
Margherita	per slice	165	692
Pepperoni	per slice	187	783
Sausage Sensations	per slice	207	866
Vege Trio	per slice	166	694
HELL PIZZA			
Desserts			
Cheesecake	per serve	506	2120
Pizza			
Brimstone	per slice	213	893
Cursed	per slice	229	957
Damned	per slice	222	930
Envy	per slice	210	878
Gluttony	per slice	201	840
Greed	per slice	215	901
Grimm	per slice	245	1030
Limbo	per slice	197	824
Lust	per slice	235	986
Mayhem	per slice	224	939
Mischief	per slice	208	872
Mordor	per slice	216	906
Nemesis	per slice	213	893
Pandemonium	per slice	240	1000
Pride	per slice	199	835
Purgatory	per slice	224	936
Serpent	per slice	262	1090
Sinister	per slice	156	653
Sloth	per slice	214	896
Temptation	per slice	224	937
Trouble	per slice	227	951
Underworld	per slice	232	972
Unearthly	per slice	229	957
Wrath	per slice	202	846
Sides			
Chicken Tenders	per serve	424	1770

FAST FOOD

	QUANTITY	CALS	KJ
Corn Nuggets	per serve	385	1610
Crumbed Camembert	per serve	655	2740
Garlic Bread	per serve	754	3160
Kumara Chips	per serve	729	3050
Lamb Shanks	per serve	986	4130
Prawn Horns	per serve	277	1160
Squid Rings	per serve	487	2040
Wedges	per serve	767	3210

KFC

Burgers

BBQ Bacon	each	479	2000
BBQ Bacon Zinger	each	573	2400
Big Snack	each	550	2300
Cheese Snack	each	426	1780
Colonel	each	377	1580
Hawaiian	each	483	2020
Hawaiian Zinger	each	583	2440
Snack	each	376	1570
Tower Burger	each	605	2530
Zinger	each	472	1980

Chicken

Chicken Nuggets, 6 pack	per serve	283	1177
Crispy Strips	2 pieces	214	892
Mini Snack Popcorn	per serve	262	1096
Original Recipe Chicken	per piece	216	902
Original Recipe Fillet	per piece	152	633
Regular Popcorn Chicken	per serve	502	2099
Wicked Wings	per piece	168	700
Zinger Fillet	per piece	219	918

Desserts

Sara Lee Choc Caramel Mousse	per serve	290	1220
Sara Lee Cookies & Cream Cheesecake	per serve	300	1254

Salads

Bean Salad	2 serves	91	380
Coleslaw, Regular	per serve	90	380

	QUANTITY	CALS	KJ
Green Side Salad	per serve	18	810
So Salad	per serve	193	810
Sides			
Bread Roll	each	120	501
Gravy, Regular	per serve	75	312
Potato & Gravy, Regular	per serve	95	97
Seasoned Chips, Regular	per serve	82	1180
Twisters & Wraps			
Crispy Chicken Wrap	each	250	1046
Pepper Mayo Twister	each	525	2200
Super Charged Twister	each	488	2040
Sweet Chilli Twister	each	445	1860
MCDONALD'S			
Beef			
Big Mac	each	494	2070
Cheeseburger	each	265	1110
Double Cheeseburger	each	443	1850
Double Quarter Pounder	each	785	3280
Grand Angus	each	630	2630
Hamburger	each	218	910
Mighty Angus	each	696	2910
Quarter Pounder	each	490	2050
Beverages			
Chocolate Shake, Medium	each	376	1570
Lime Shake, Medium	each	318	1330
Strawberry Shake, Medium	each	345	1440
Breakfast			
Bacon & Egg McMuffin	each	305	1280
BLT Bagel	each	354	1480
Egg, Tomato & Bacon Wrap	each	387	1620
English Brekkie Wrap	each	493	2060
Hashbrown	each	153	640
Hotcakes	each	329	1370
Kellogg's Just Right Original Cereal	per serve	160	670
Kellogg's Nutri-Grain Cereal Bowl	per serve	114	479

FAST FOOD

	QUANTITY	CALS	KJ
Kiwi Big Breakfast	each	675	2820
Massive McMuffin	each	546	2280
NYC Benedict	each	394	1990
Sausage & Egg McMuffin	each	386	1610
Sausage McMuffin	each	300	1260
Toasted Bagel with Jam & Whipped Butter	each	330	1380
Toasted English Muffin	each	151	631
Chicken & Fish			
Chick McBites	each	158	661
Chick'n McCheese	each	341	1420
Chicken McNuggets, 3 pack	per serve	134	564
Chicken 'n' Mayo Burger	each	353	1480
Chicken Tenders, 3 pack	per serve	326	1360
Crispy Chicken Ciabatta, Tangy BBQ	each	704	2940
Crispy Chicken Ciabatta, Zesto Mayo	each	710	2970
Filet-O-Fish	each	319	1330
McChamp Chicken Burger	each	527	2200
McChicken	each	367	1530
McGrilled Chicken Burger	each	453	1900
McSpicy Chicken Burger	each	523	2190
Desserts			
Birthday Party Chocolate Cake	each	218	911
Flake Cone	each	187	780
Hot Apple Pie	each	236	985
McFlurry, Bubblegum Squash	each	278	1160
McFlurry, M&M Minis	each	393	1640
McFlurry, Oreo	each	310	1300
Soft Serve Cone	each	141	591
Sundae, Caramel, Small	each	343	1430
Sundae, Hot Fudge, Small	each	336	1400
Sundae, Strawberry, Small	each	275	1150
Georgie Pie			
Chicken 'N' Vegetable Pie	each	518	2170
Steak Mince 'N' Cheese Pie	each	567	2370

	QUANTITY	CALS	KJ
McWraps			
Crispy Chicken & Aioli	each	641	2680
Crispy Chicken & Honey Soy	each	644	2690
Crispy Chicken Snack	each	275	1150
Crispy Chicken Spicy Mayo	each	644	2690
Grilled Chicken & Aioli	each	557	2330
Grilled Chicken & Honey Soy	each	533	2230
Grilled Chicken Snack	each	234	976
Grilled Chicken Spicy Mayo	each	560	2340
Salad & Fruit			
Crispy Noodle Crispy Chicken Salad	each	361	1510
Crispy Noodle Grilled Chicken Salad	each	274	1150
Fruit Bag	each	41	174
Garden Salad	each	15	70
Warm Crispy Chicken Salad	each	261	1090
Warm Grilled Chicken Salad	each	176	737
Sides, French Fries, Medium	per serve	330	1380
NANDO'S			
¼ Chicken, Breast, With Skin	each	345	1447
¼ Chicken, Breast, Without Skin	each	281	1178
Chicken Burger, With Mayo	each	436	1828
Chicken Burger, Without Mayo	each	399	1673
Grilled Chicken Salad, With Dressing	per serve	156	656
Grilled Chicken Salad, Without Dressing	per serve	132	556
Individual Chicken Rib	each	49	206
Pita, With Mayo	each	353	1477
Pita, Without Mayo	each	314	1316
Regular Chips	per serve	466	1950
Regular Spicy Rice	per serve	203	853
PIZZA HUT			
Classic, Large			
Apricot Chicken	per slice	173	730
BBQ Chicken & Bacon	per slice	188	790
Beef & Onion	per slice	174	730
Beef Italiano	per slice	205	860

FAST FOOD

	QUANTITY	CALS	KJ
Cheese Extreme	per slice	208	870
Classic Italian	per slice	191	800
Ham & Cheese	per slice	187	790
Hawaiian	per slice	190	800
Hot & Spicy	per slice	202	850
Meat Lovers	per slice	207	870
Mexican Veg Supreme	per slice	106	710
Mushroom & Cheese	per slice	170	720
Pepperoni	per slice	183	770
Satay Chicken	per slice	186	780
Seafood Deluxe	per slice	198	830
Super Supreme	per slice	202	850
Veg Delight	per slice	146	610
Deep Pan, Large			
Apricot Chicken	per slice	196	820
BBQ Chicken & Bacon	per slice	200	840
Beef & Onion	per slice	200	840
Beef Italiano	per slice	216	910
Cheese Extreme	per slice	220	920
Classic Italian	per slice	216	910
Ham & Cheese	per slice	200	840
Hawaiian	per slice	215	900
Hot & Spicy	per slice	230	950
Meat Lovers	per slice	218	920
Mexican Veg Supreme	per slice	174	765
Mushroom & Cheese	per slice	181	760
Pepperoni	per slice	195	820
Satay Chicken	per slice	198	830
Seafood Deluxe	per slice	210	880
Super Supreme	per slice	228	960
Veg Delight	per slice	144	600
Sides			
Cheesy Garlic Bread	4 slices	666	2787
Chicken Wings	5 wings	488	2039
Foccacia Breadsticks	5 pieces	616	2576

	QUANTITY	CALS	KJ
Fries	per serve	603	2519
Garlic Bread	2 slices	167	700
Stuffed Crust			
Apricot Chicken	per slice	201	840
BBQ Chicken & Bacon	per slice	227	948
Beef & Onion	per slice	202	850
Beef Italiano	per slice	233	980
Cheese Extreme	per slice	203	847
Classic Italian	per slice	219	920
Hawaiian	per slice	216	910
Ham & Cheese	per slice	204	850
Hot & Spicy	per slice	228	960
Meat Lovers	per slice	222	930
Mexican Veg Supreme	per slice	202	884
Mushroom & Cheese	per slice	198	830
Pepperoni	per slice	214	900
Satay Chicken	per slice	213	890
Seafood Deluxe	per slice	212	890
Super Supreme	per slice	229	960
Veg Delight	per slice	147	620
Thin & Crispy, Large			
Apricot Chicken	per slice	173	730
BBQ Chicken & Bacon	per slice	137	570
Beef & Onion	per slice	136	570
Beef Italiano	per slice	167	700
Cheese Extreme	per slice	171	720
Classic Italian	per slice	153	640
Ham & Cheese	per slice	137	570
Hawaiian	per slice	154	640
Hot & Spicy	per slice	163	680
Meat Lovers	per slice	169	710
Mexican Veg Supreme	per slice	149	624
Mushroom & Cheese	per slice	132	550
Pepperoni	per slice	148	620
Satay Chicken	per slice	146	610

FAST FOOD

	QUANTITY	CALS	KJ
Seafood Deluxe	per slice	159	670
Super Supreme	per slice	164	690
Veg Delight	per slice	110	440
SUBWAY			
6-inch Breakfast Sandwiches			
Bacon, Egg & Cheese	each	318	1330
Egg & Cheese	each	311	1300
Ham, Egg & Cheese	each	298	1250
Sausage, Egg & Cheese	each	425	1780
Steak, Egg & Cheese	each	331	1380
Western Egg & Cheese	each	292	1220
6-inch Flatbread Sandwiches			
Chicken Strips	each	350	1460
Chicken Teriyaki	each	383	1600
Ham	each	333	1390
Oven Roasted Chicken	each	382	1600
Roast Beef	each	337	1410
Subway Club	each	343	1440
Turkey	each	327	1370
Turkey & Ham	each	338	1410
Veggie Delight	each	282	1180
6-inch Subs			
Chicken & Bacon Ranch Melt	each	456	1910
Chicken Classic	each	334	1400
Chicken Strips	each	275	1150
Chicken Teriyaki	each	308	1290
Ham	each	258	1080
Italian BMT	each	335	1400
Meatball Marinara	each	363	1520
Oven Roasted Chicken	each	307	1290
Pizza Sub	each	362	1520
Pork Riblet	each	437	1830
Roast Beef	each	262	1100
Seafood Sensation	each	292	1220
Steak & Cheese	each	343	1440

	QUANTITY	CALS	KJ
Subway Club	each	269	1120
Subway Melt	each	347	1450
Tuna	each	266	1110
Turkey	each	253	1060
Turkey & Ham	each	263	1100
Veggie Delite	each	207	867
Veggie Patty	each	397	1660
Breakfast Omelettes			
Bacon, Egg & Cheese	each	132	552
Egg & Cheese	each	125	525
French Toast	each	233	974
Ham, Egg & Cheese	each	112	469
Sausage, Egg & Cheese	each	239	1100
Steak, Egg & Cheese	each	184	768
Western Egg & Cheese	each	138	774
Cookies			
Chocolate Chip	each	208	872
Double Chocolate Chip	each	212	887
M&Ms	each	204	852
Oat & Raisin	each	185	775
White Chip Macadamia Nut	each	219	916
Mini Subs			
Ham	each	163	683
Roast Beef	each	174	729
Tuna	each	167	699
Turkey	each	168	703
Veggie Delite	each	138	576
Salads			
Ham	each	109	456
Roast Beef	each	113	471
Roasted Chicken	each	126	526
Subway Club	each	119	499
Sweet Onion Chicken Teriyaki	each	158	663
Turkey	each	103	432
Turkey & Ham	each	114	476

	QUANTITY	CALS	KJ
Veggie Delite	each	58	242
Sides			
Apple Slices	each	42	177
Yoghurt	each	136	568
Wraps			
Chicken Teriyaki	each	313	1350
Ham	each	267	1150
Roast Beef	each	267	1150
Roasted Chicken	each	283	1220
Subway Club	each	276	1190
Turkey	each	261	1130
Turkey & Ham	each	271	1170
Veggie Delite	each	215	938
WENDY'S			
Baked Potatoes			
Bacon & Cheese	each	440	1247
Chili & Cheese	each	448	1874
Mushroom & Cheese	each	282	1179
Plain	each	234	978
Sour Cream & Chives	each	339	1419
Breakfast			
Bacon Avocado Muffin	each	298	1136
Bacon, Egg & Cheese Muffin	each	269	1125
Breakfast Baconator Muffin	each	436	1823
Breakfast Mushroom Melt	each	436	1823
Breakfast Platter	each	437	1831
Country Muffin	each	367	1535
Mince & Beans on Toast	each	294	1233
Pancakes	each	430	1801
Burgers			
¼lb Single	each	458	1919
½lb Double	each	694	2908
¾lb Triple	each	931	3896
Avocado Bacon Supreme	each	607	2541
Bacon Cheeseburger	each	358	1501

	QUANTITY	CALS	KJ
Baconater	each	771	3226
Baconater Mushroom Melt	each	785	3284
Big Bacon Classic	each	562	2351
Cheeseburger	each	368	1330
Chicken Club	each	618	2589
Crispy Chicken	each	420	1757
Deluxe Cheeseburger	each	349	1462
Hamburger	each	328	1163
Hoki	each	329	1377
Homestyle Chicken	each	537	2247
Kid Meal, Cheeseburger	each	309	1294
Kid Meal, Hamburger	each	269	1127
Spicy Chicken	each	507	2125
Ultimate Chicken Grill	each	412	1723
Desserts			
Frosty Cone, Small	each	222	929
Oreo Parfait	each	330	1382
Wild Berry Pancakes	per serve	307	1285
Salads			
Mandarin Chicken, Base	each	180	755
Side, No Dressing	each	58	244
Taco, Base	each	424	1776
Side Orders			
Chicken Nuggets, 5 pieces	per serve	231	968
Chili, Small	each	257	1076
Chili Guacamole Fries	per serve	662	2770
French Fries, Medium	each	387	1622
Guacamole Crunch Bowl	per serve	618	2589
Loaded Cheese Fries	per serve	392	1639

Fish

Albacore Tuna	100g	70	293
Alfonsino	100g	120	502
Anchovy Fillets	100g	156	656

FISH

	QUANTITY	CALS	KJ
Barracuda	100g	140	586
Baxter's Dogfish	100g	100	419
Black Oreo Dory	100g	71	297
Black Slickhead	100g	57	238
Blue Cod	100g	102	427
Blue Mackerel	100g	100	420
Blue Moki	100g	123	515
Bluff Oysters	100g	123	515
Calamari Chips	100g	119	498
Cardinal	100g	113	473
Caviar	100g	100	420
Cockles, *boiled*	100g	39	161
Crab, *raw*	100g	84	351
Crayfish/Lobster	100g	82	343
Eel, *smoked*	100g	167	699
Fish, *fried in batter*	100g	228	953
Fish Cakes	100g	193	805
Fish Chowder	1 cup	240	1005
Fish Fillets, *baked*	100g	212	885
Fish Fingers	each	50	209
Fish Nuggets	6 nuggets	210	878
Flounder, *baked*	100g	126	524
Garfish (Piper)	100g	118	494
Gemfish	100g	130	544
Giant Stargazer (Monkfish)	100g	100	419
Green Mussel	100g	95	398
Grenadier (Rattail)	100g	100	419
Grey Mullet (Striped)	100g	117	489
Grouper	per piece	165	691
Hake	100g	71	298
Hapuku	100g	119	498
Hoki			
baked	100g	101	421
deep-fried	100g	172	717
Jack Mackerel	100g	69	289

	QUANTITY	CALS	KJ
Kahawai			
baked	100g	131	546
deep-fried	100g	185	775
Kina (Sea Egg)	1 tbsp	13	55
Kingfish			
fresh	100g	123	515
smoked	100g	98	410
Kippered Herrings	100g	217	907
Leatherjacket	100g	104	435
Lemon Sole	2 fillets	387	1619
Ling	100g	87	364
Lookdown Dory	100g	122	511
Moreton Bay Bugs	100g	92	385
Mussels			
marinated	100g	129	537
smoked	100g	197	823
steamed	100g	120	498
New Zealand Sole	100g	112	469
Octopus, raw	100g	82	343
Orange Roughy			
baked	100g	175	730
deep-fried	100g	191	797
Oysters			
fried in batter	100g	228	950
raw	100g	93	390
Paddle Crab	100g	93	389
Pale Ghost Shark	100g	101	423
Parore	100g	112	469
Paua (Abalone)	100g	105	439
Paua Fritter, deep-fried	100g	261	1090
Peppered Mackerel	100g	158	662
Pilchards, tinned in tomato sauce	100g	125	523
Pipis, raw	100g	41	172
Prawns/Shrimps	100g	99	414
Ray's Bream	100g	123	515

FISH

	QUANTITY	CALS	KJ
Red Cod	100g	96	402
Red Gurnard	100g	111	465
Ribaldo	100g	98	410
Ridge-scaled Rattail	100g	96	402
Rig (Lemonfish)	100g	120	502
Rudderfish	100g	241	1009
Salmon			
caviar	20g	11	46
freshwater	100g	129	540
sea pen	100g	166	695
smoked	100g	133	558
Sardines, *tinned*	100g	218	913
Scallops			
fresh	100g	88	368
fried in batter	100g	209	871
Sea Perch	100g	88	368
Shrimps, *tinned*	100g	94	393
Silver Dory	100g	101	423
Silver Warehou	100g	198	829
Skipjack Tuna	100g	103	431
Slender Tuna	100g	326	1365
Snapper			
baked	100g	133	556
deep-fried	100g	154	643
Southern Blue Whiting	100g	89	372
Spiny Dogfish	100g	223	933
Squid Rings, *fried*	100g	239	999
Tarakihi			
baked	100g	111	461
deep-fried	100g	139	579
Trevally	100g	130	544
Trout, *raw*	100g	148	619
Tuna	100g	141	589
White Warehou	100g	190	796

	QUANTITY	CALS	KJ
Whitebait			
fresh	125g	39	163
pattie	each	58	243
Yellow-Eyed Mullet	100g	114	477

From the Deli

	QUANTITY	CALS	KJ
Beef Pastrami	28g	41	171
Falafel Ball, *fried*	100g	195	814
Salad			
Greek	100g	36	151
Potato	100g	147	612
Rice	100g	86	356
Samosa, Vegetable	100g	196	716
Tabbouleh	100g	57	234
ALWAYS FRESH			
Dolmades	60g	93	392
Eggplant, Char-grilled	50g	51	216
Mixed Olives	70g	127	535
Piquillo Peppers	50g	17	75
ARISTOCRAT			
Pickled Onions	25g	15	63
Spiced Gherkins	25g	17	70
BEEHIVE			
Shaved Champagne Ham	100g	90	379
Shaved Chicken Breast	100g	91	383
Shaved Honey Baked Ham	100g	94	397
Shaved Peppered Ham	100g	79	331
Shaved Seasoned Ham	100g	90	379
Sliced Honey Baked Ham	100g	94	397
BROOKS DELI			
Biersticks, all flavours	100g	351	1470
Salami Slices			
Cracked Pepper	100g	351	1470
Dutch	100g	351	1470

FROM THE DELI

	QUANTITY	CALS	KJ
Garlica	100g	351	1470
Italiano	100g	351	1470
Italiano, Reduced Fat	100g	256	1070
Pepperoni	100g	351	1470
Pepperoni, Reduced Fat	100g	256	1070
Snyworst	100g	351	1470
Salami Sticks, all flavours	100g	351	1470
DELMAINE			
Baby Gherkins	100g	32	135
Caperberries	15g	3	16
Capers	15g	4	19
Chargrilled Artichokes	30g	44	188
Chargrilled Capsicum	50g	14	60
Chargrilled Eggplant	30g	35	146
Chargrilled Red Capsicum	40g	30	126
Gherkins	36g	11	48
Green Peppercorns	8g	35	234
Jalapeños	30g	4	20
Long Sliced Gherkins	100g	32	134
Marinated Artichoke Hearts	32g	60	251
Marinated Feta	28g	75	314
Marinated Feta & Sundried Tomatoes	26g	39	165
Mediterranean Mix	100g	213	892
Olives			
Almond Stuffed	15g	31	130
Jumbo Kalamata	100g	237	995
Kalamata Balsamic & Rosemary	12g	32	134
Kalamata Wedges	15g	41	174
Marinated Black Olives	40g	106	445
Mixed Green & Black	40g	95	399
Olive Grove Selection	40g	77	324
Pimento Stuffed Green	15g	21	87
Pitted Black	15g	18	78
Pitted Colossal Green	15g	21	88
Pitted Jumbo Kalamata	15g	35	149

	QUANTITY	CALS	KJ
Plain Green	15g	27	116
Queen Green Feta & Ricotta	15g	59	251
Queen Green Stuffed with Garlic	10g	13	53
Sliced Black	15g	19	83
Stuffed Green	15g	27	123
Pickled Onions	5g	13	55
Round Sliced Gherkins	36g	32	134
Silverskin Onions	100g	23	99
Sundried Tomatoes in Oil	29g	62	261
Sundried Tomatoes in Water	40g	38	161
FREEDOM FARMS			
Boneless Leg Ham	100g	92	388
Champagne Ham	100g	133	559
Ham on the Bone	100g	172	722
Shaved Manuka Honey Leg Ham	100g	99	418
Shaved NZ Champagne Ham	100g	90	379
HELLERS			
Angus Peppered Roast Beef	100g	118	496
Bacon Strips	100g	107	451
Champagne Leg Ham	100g	162	678
Continental Deli Meats			
Devilled Beef	100g	126	530
Devilled Pork	100g	126	530
Pastrami	100g	127	535
Polish Sausage	100g	212	890
Roast Beef	100g	124	520
Cooked Silverside	100g	126	531
Honey Baked Ham	100g	107	450
Hot Pork	100g	174	730
Manuka Smoked Leg Ham	100g	107	451
Mild Biersticks	100g	300	1259
Pizza Salami	100g	239	1000
Roast Chicken	100g	131	550
Seasoned Pastrami	100g	105	440
Smoked Beef	100g	121	510

FROM THE DELI

	QUANTITY	CALS	KJ
Smoked Chicken	100g	88	370
Spicy Biersticks	100g	302	1267
SWISS DELI			
Cold Cuts & Loaves			
Balleron	100g	220	919
Beer Loaf	100g	169	707
Berne Lyoner	100g	219	915
Bierwurst	100g	188	785
Cold Cuts	100g	220	919
Garlic Roll	100g	207	864
Ham Roll	100g	171	717
Mortadella	100g	206	862
Mushroom Lyoner	100g	219	915
Veal & Pork Loaf	100g	224	936
Vienna Roll	100g	227	949
Continentals & Salamis			
Air Dried Beef	100g	163	683
Continental Speck	100g	342	1432
Kassler	100g	116	485
Landjaeger	100g	376	1574
Pantli	100g	376	1574
Pastrami	100g	100	417
Pork Brawn	100g	113	472
Salametti Lugano	100g	336	1405
Salami, Alpine	100g	364	1522
Salami, Dutch	100g	341	1426
Salami, Italian	100g	356	1489
Snackies	100g	303	1266
Hams			
Champagne	100g	159	664
Double Smoked	100g	155	650
Farm Smoked	100g	114	478
Ham on Bone	100g	150	626
Pressed	100g	110	461
Supreme Leg	100g	111	463

	QUANTITY	CALS	KJ
TEGEL			
Chicken Cocktail Sausage	100g	195	818
Chicken Luncheon	100g	200	837
Classic Sliced Roast Chicken	100g	91	382
Deli Fresh			
Lime & Coriander Tenderloins	100g	116	487
Roast Garlic Chicken Breast	100g	116	489
Honey Roast Sliced Turkey	100g	101	423
Meal Maker			
Diced Roast Chicken	100g	133	559
Sliced Roast Chicken	100g	134	563
Shredded Roast Chicken	100g	131	550
Original Manuka Smoked Chicken Bacon	100g	99	416
Shaved Kamahi Honey Chicken	100g	87	367
Shaved Manuka Smoked Chicken	100g	87	367
Shredded Italian Herb Chicken	100g	131	550
Shredded Roast Chicken	100g	129	541
Smokehouse Honey Whole Chicken	100g	169	709
Smokehouse Sweet Chilli Breast	100g	114	480
Smokehouse Traditional Whole Chicken	100g	154	646
Thick Cut Manuka Smoked Chicken Bacon	100g	99	416
VERKERKS			
Beef & Garlic Kranksy	100g	241	1010
Bier Sticks, Dutch Spice Blend	100g	236	990
Cabanossi Sticks, European Spice Blend	100g	236	989
Chorizo Sticks, Spanish Spice Blend	100g	242	1014
Frankfurters	100g	203	852
Hot Pork	100g	191	801
Original Kranksy	100g	225	945
Pastrami	100g	98	411
Prosciutto	100g	224	939
Rookworst	100g	241	1010
Salami			

	QUANTITY	CALS	KJ
Dutch	100g	276	1155
Italian	100g	275	1154
Lean Danish	100g	154	646
Lean Italian	100g	188	788
Lean Pepperoni	100g	201	843
Pepperoni	100g	276	1155

From the Freezer

Frozen Meals

AASHIAYANA

Butter Chicken	100g	132	552
Chicken Tikka Masala	100g	125	525
Lamb Korma	100g	185	774
Lamb Rogan Josh	100g	134	559
Thali	100g	150	627
ANDREW CORBETT			
BB Grillers	100g	193	802
Chargrilled Cooked Patties	100g	198	829
Meteors Meat Patties	100g	193	802
ANGEL BAY			
Gluten Free Burger Patties	100g	225	944
Gourmet Cheese Beef Burger Patties	100g	288	1209
Gourmet Lamb Nuggets	100g	215	900
Gourmet Lite Beef Bites	100g	391	636
Lite Beef Burger Patties	100g	391	636
Super Gourmet Beef Burger Patties	100g	236	991
ARIA FARM			
Beef Strips	100g	195	820
Lamb Strips	100g	183	769
AUNT BETTY'S, Yorkshire Pudding	100g	309	1293
BIRDS EYE			
Bubble 'n Squeak	100g	207	867
Corn Fritters	100g	210	881
Vegetable Fingers	100g	194	813

	QUANTITY	CALS	KJ
Salmon Cakes with Veges	100g	199	834
CORBIES, Beef Patties	100g	176	736
DAKSHIN'S			
Butter Chicken	100g	214	899
Chicken Tikka Masala	100g	143	602
Rogan Josh	100g	149	625
Thai Green Curry	100g	141	594
FRANKLIN, Beef Patties	100g	188	788
IRVINES			
Super Snack			
Beef Lasagne	100g	107	450
Butter Chicken	100g	360	576
Homestyle Cottage Pie	100g	120	503
Homestyle Fish Pie	100g	102	430
Macaroni Cheese	100g	439	620
Mild Beef Curry	100g	111	465
MCCAIN			
Chicken Parmagiana	100g	144	600
Healthy Choice			
Beef Florentine	100g	89	372
Cottage Pie	100g	88	365
Lasagne	100g	148	618
Singapore Noodles with Chicken	100g	89	371
Roast Chicken	100g	87	364
Roast Lamb	100g	98	409
Shepherd's Pie	100g	101	424
Veal Cordon Bleu	100g	157	654
PAMS			
Chunky Cut Fries	100g	132	554
Crinkle Cut Fries	100g	141	592
Crunchy Wedges	100g	122	512
Mashed Potatoes	100g	102	427
Mini Hash Browns	100g	166	698
Potato Balls	100g	167	702

FROM THE FREEZER

	QUANTITY	CALS	KJ
Sausage Rolls			
Cheese	100g	243	1020
Original	100g	255	1070
Shoestring Fries	100g	159	669
Straight Cut Fries	100g	132	553
QUORN			
Chicken-Style & Mushroom Pastries	100g	259	1080
Classic Burgers	100g	155	650
Meat-Style Balls	100g	102	426
Mince	100g	103	434
Pieces	100g	98	411
Sausages	100g	129	543
Schnitzel, Cheese & Spinach	100g	223	936
SHORE MARINER			
Mini Hot Dogs	100g	211	886
Onion Bhajis	100g	162	679
Vegetable Pakoras	100g	202	846
Vegetable Samosas	100g	172	721
Vegetable Spring Rolls	100g	24	104
SIGNATURE RANGE			
Beef Lasagne	100g	139	583
Chicken & Mushroom Risotto	100g	101	423
Chicken & White Wine	100g	121	504
Macaroni Cheese	100g	156	651
WATTIE'S			
Beef Lasagne	100g	100	420
Butter Chicken	100g	127	535
Cheesy Bacon Pasta	100g	138	580
Chicken Chow Mein	100g	89	375
Chicken Fried Rice	100g	113	475
Chilli Con Carne	100g	103	435
Cordon Bleu	100g	130	545
Cottage Pie	100g	127	535
Fish Pie	100g	108	455
Macaroni Cheese	100g	157	660

	QUANTITY	CALS	KJ
Roast Beef	100g	103	435
Roast Chicken	100g	109	460
Roast Lamb	100g	84	355
Roast Pork	100g	78	330
Sweet & Sour Pork	100g	113	475
WEIGHT WATCHERS			
Beef Burgundy	100g	49	200
Beef Cannelloni	100g	90	380
Beef Hot Pot	100g	63	265
Beef Lasagne	100g	95	400
Butter Chicken	100g	118	495
Chicken Fettucine	100g	101	425
Chicken Pesto Spaghettini	100g	113	475
Chicken Risotto	100g	97	410
Chicken Tikka Masala	100g	84	355
Cottage Pie	100g	81	340
Country Chicken Casserole	100g	62	260
Creamy Chicken & Mushroom Risotto	100g	99	415
Creamy Garlic Prawns	100g	101	425
Creamy Mushroom Risotto	100g	97	410
Thai Chicken Curry	100g	105	440
Tuna Bake	100g	96	405
Frozen Potato Products			
BIRDS EYE			
Golden Crunch Beer Battered Chips	100g	107	450
Golden Crunch Hash Browns	100g	175	733
Golden Crunch Potato Gems	100g	152	639
Hash Browns	100g	175	733
KAURI COAST KUMARA			
Chips	100g	150	629
Rosti	100g	97	827
Rosti, Spinach, Feta & Garlic	100g	169	708
MCCAIN			
Beer Batter			
Chunky	100g	151	632

FROM THE FREEZER

	QUANTITY	CALS	KJ
Shoestring	100g	183	764
Steak Cut Fries	100g	158	662
Wedges	100g	151	633
Mini Roast Potatoes			
Italian Herbs	100g	132	550
Sea Salt & Garlic	100g	132	551
Potato Snacks, Hash Browns	100g	169	705
Seasoned Fries & Wedges			
Curly Fries	100g	187	782
Hot Bandito Potato Wedges	125g	188	784
Original Wedges	125g	188	784
Superfries			
Chunky Cut	100g	124	517
Original	100g	163	680
Shoestring	100g	162	677
Straight Cut	100g	138	576
WATTIE'S			
Fries & Wedges			
Chunky Cut Golden Chips	100g	132	555
Crispy Crinkles	100g	141	590
Crispy Skins	100g	138	580
Crunchy Beer Batter Steak Cut Fries	100g	146	615
Jacket Wedges	100g	121	510
Kumara Fries	100g	149	625
Shoestring Fries	100g	160	670
Super Oven Golden Chips	100g	132	555
Hash Browns			
Classic	100g	172	720
Pom Poms	100g	190	795
Tri-browns, Classic	100g	162	680
Potato Roasters			
Rosemary & Garlic	100g	143	600
Southern Style	100g	138	580

	QUANTITY	CALS	KJ
Frozen Poultry			
INGHAM			
Breast Tenders, Original	100g	187	785
Breast Tenders, Sweet Chilli	100g	219	917
Cordon Bleu, Ham & Cheese	100g	195	818
Kiev, Garlic Butter	100g	262	1100
TEGEL			
Chargrill-style Chicken Steaks	each	168	706
Chicken Nuggets			
Battered	120g	232	971
Bites	150g	302	1266
Chinese Honey Bites	150g	325	1361
Crumbed	120g	226	947
Crumbed Burgers	100g	202	849
Zoo Animals	130g	247	1036
Cuisine			
Apricot & Cream Cheese	100g	184	771
Cordon Bleu	100g	188	790
Crumbed Tender Loins	100g	185	777
Garlic Kiev	100g	189	793
Parmigiana Schnitzel	100g	190	796
Party Bites			
BBQ Chicken	100g	168	704
Buffalo Chicken	100g	189	794
Southern Style Chicken	100g	187	786
Ready to Roast with Apricot Stuffing	150g	267	1119
Real Deal			
Chicken Hot Dogs	each	230	966
Chicken Loopys	100g	211	885
Chicken Nuggets	100g	229	959
Hawaiian Filled Breasts	each	215	901
Spicy Crumb Burgers	each	137	577
Southern Style Nibbles	100g	317	1329
Take Outs			
Flame Grilled Original Chicken Steaks	each	167	701

FROM THE FREEZER

	QUANTITY	CALS	KJ
Flame Grilled Thai Chicken Steaks	each	163	686
Golden Crumb Chicken Schnitzel	each	226	946
Original Crispy Crumb Chicken Tenders	150g	269	1128
Frozen Seafood			
BIRDS EYE			
Oven Bake			
Crumbed	100g	209	878
Herb & Garlic	100g	209	878
Lemon	100g	209	878
Lemon Pepper	100g	226	949
Lightly Battered	100g	227	952
PACIFIC WEST, Beer Battered Snapper Fillets	100g	162	678
SEALORD			
Cafe Style Fish Cakes			
Classic	100g	132	555
Potato & Leek	100g	158	663
Calamari Chips	100g	25	106
Dory, Wholemeal Crumb	100g	183	769
Fish Fingers, Oat Crumb	100g	195	816
Hoki Bites	100g	175	735
Hoki, Beer Batter	100g	214	898
Hoki, Classic Crumb	100g	161	675
Hoki, Garlic Sauce	100g	192	804
Hoki, Lemon Pepper Crumb	100g	182	763
Hoki, Parsley Sauce	100g	196	824
Hoki, Tempura Batter	100g	214	898
Hoki Fillets	100g	83	349
Hoki Fillets, Beer Battered with Stoke	100g	146	613
Hoki Fillets, Crunchy Crumb	100g	181	760
Hoki Fillets, Sweet Chilli	100g	190	795
Hoki Fillets, Tomato & Italian Herb	100g	201	842
Hoki Fillets with Linseed, Sunflower & Pumpkin Seeds	100g	170	715
Hoki Fillets with Wholemeal	100g	187	783

	QUANTITY	CALS	KJ
Hoki Tapas			
Kumara Crumb	100g	186	779
Sweet Chilli Crumb	100g	191	801
Orange Roughy	100g	68	288
Orange Roughy, Wholemeal Crumb	100g	218	913
WAITOA			
Ancient Grains	100g	173	727
Original Tenders	100g	187	785
Tempura Nuggets	100g	181	757
Frozen Snacks			
BORG'S			
Spinach & Ricotta Cheese Pastizzi	100g	226	948
Spinach & Ricotta Cheese Triangles	100g	280	1170
Vegetarian Triangles	100g	227	950
HIGHMARK			
Mini Spring Rolls	100g	244	1020
Spring Rolls, Chicken Noodle	100g	220	920
Spring Rolls, Traditional Beef	100g	246	824
Wontons, Pork	100g	277	950
HO MAI			
Cocktail Spring Roll	100g	221	927
Mini Dim Sim, Beef	100g	201	844
HOMEBRAND			
Pork & Chinese Dumpling	100g	238	996
Sausage Rolls	100g	264	1105
Spring Roll	100g	246	1030
NEWWAY, Chicken Sausage Rolls	100g	209	878
SIGNATURE RANGE			
Cheese Sausage Rolls	100g	275	1150
Sausage Rolls	100g	238	1080
Frozen Vegetables			
HOMEBRAND			
Green Beans	100g	34	145
Mixed Vegetables	100g	55	230
Peas	100g	81	340

FROM THE FREEZER

	QUANTITY	CALS	KJ
MAMASAN, Shelled Edamame Soybeans	100g	158	665
MCCAIN			
Baby Beans, Baby Carrots & Peas	100g	44	185
Baby Minted Peas	100g	76	319
Baby Peas	100g	72	300
Beans, Sliced	100g	35	147
Broccoli	100g	29	122
Brussels Sprouts	100g	51	215
Carrots, Cauliflower, Broccoli & Peas	100g	26	111
Corn Cobettes	100g	95	397
Corn, Super Juicy	100g	93	390
Garden Greens	100g	66	369
Mixed Veges	100g	80	334
Peas	100g	89	373
Peas & Super Juicy Corn Kernels	100g	93	387
Peas, Corn & Carrot	100g	80	334
Peas, Mint	100g	88	369
Stir-fry Supreme Veges	100g	33	136
Winter Veges	100g	31	128
SELECT			
Baby Peas	100g	73	306
Broad Beans	100g	80	333
Cauliflower & Broccoli Florets	100g	28	117
Eastern Stir-fry	100g	37	156
Garden Stir-fry	100g	67	280
Peas, Carrots & Corn	100g	67	280
Whole Green Beans	100g	35	145
Winter Vegetable Mix	100g	42	117
SIGNATURE RANGE			
Supersweet Corn Kernels	100g	79	332
Whole Baby Carrots	100g	40	168
TALLEYS			
Garden Peas	100g	65	273
Mixed Vegetables	100g	73	309
Spinach Portions	100g	24	102

	QUANTITY	CALS	KJ
WATTIE'S			
Baby Peas	100g	69	290
Baby Peas & Super Sweet Corn	100g	76	320
Broccoli & Cauliflower Medley	100g	27	115
Choice Cut Green Beans	100g	25	105
Chopped Spinach	100g	45	190
Chunky Mix	100g	28	120
Corn			
Chuckwagon	100g	65	275
Supersweet	100g	88	370
Supersweet Corn Cobs	100g	88	370
Garden Peas	100g	86	360
Minted Garden Peas	100g	86	360
Mixed Vegetables	100g	52	220
Peas & Corn	100g	87	365
Rainbow Mix	100g	40	170
SteamFresh			
Broccoli, Carrots & Sugar Snap Peas	100g	33	140
Carrots, Broccoli & Cauliflower	100g	28	120
Carrots, Supersweet Corn & Sugarsnap Peas	100g	52	220
Supersweet Corn, Carrots & Broccoli	100g	51	215
Stir-Fry Mix			
7 Veges	100g	46	195
Chinese	100g	27	115
International	100g	27	115
Stir-fry Mix for Sweet & Sour	100g	29	125
Super Greens	100g	51	215
Super Mix	100g	27	115
Wok Creations			
Chinese Style	100g	29	125
Hong Kong	100g	31	130
Malaysian	100g	51	215

	QUANTITY	CALS	KJ

From the Fridge

Dip, Hummus, Pâté, Pesto & Salsa

BRETON

Pâté

Chicken & Port	10g	33	141
Cracked Pepper	10g	30	127
French Herb	10g	31	131
Garlic	10g	31	132

COUNTRY GOODNESS

Dip

Cheese & Onion	20g	32	134
Green Onion	20g	30	125
Kiwi Onion	20g	31	128
Seafood Fiesta	20g	30	126
Sour Cream & Chives	20g	30	126

DELMAINE

Dip

Artichoke & Red Pepper Bruschetta	30g	46	196
Artichoke Bruschetta	30g	49	208
Asparagus Bruschetta	30g	49	209
Red Pepper & Jalapeno Bruschetta	30g	34	146

Pesto

Basil with Extra Parmesan	10g	47	198
Traditional Basil	10g	46	196
DOLMIO, Pesto, Traditional Basil	40g	53	225
FOOD BY CHEFS, Basil Pesto	25g	115	485

GENOESE

Chunky Pesto Dip	100g	573	2400
Pesto, Fresh Basil	100g	448	2087

JUST HUMMUS

Garlic & Lemon	100g	168	705
Roasted Carrot & Honey	100g	248	1040
Roasted Kumara	100g	148	620

	QUANTITY	CALS	KJ
LISA'S			
Dip			
Aubergine & Cashew with Coriander & Lime	20g	87	362
Mexican Chipotle Salsa	20g	35	145
Moroccan Carrot with Cumin & Coriander	20g	41	172
Pumpkin & Kumara with Roast Cashew & Cumin	20g	41	171
Roasted Kumara with Orange & Mint	20g	46	192
Feta & Baby Spinach with Black Pepper	20g	49	204
Feta & Basil with Crushed Garlic	20g	58	244
Feta & Caramelised Onion with a hint of Basil	20g	58	244
Hummus			
Caramelised Onion with Lemon & Raspberry	20g	57	240
Gloriously Garlic	20g	75	315
Grilled Capsicum with Lemon & Tahini	20g	59	250
Jalapeno & Lime with Coriander	20g	53	221
Original with Garlic & Lemon	20g	45	191
Sundried Tomato with Fresh Basil	20g	46	193
Toppings			
Almond Dukkah with Sesame & Chilli on Smooth Hummus	20g	77	321
Coriander Pesto on Kumara Hummus	20g	65	272
Harissa with Roast Red Pepper on Pumpkin Hummus	20g	47	196
Hummus with Dukkah & Roasted Pistachio	20g	84	350
Hummus with Roasted Garlic	20g	79	331
Hummus with Sundried Tomato Pesto	20g	76	318
Kumara with Crunchy Pumpkin Seeds	20g	72	300
Masala Dukkah on Pumpkin Hummus	20g	69	290

FROM THE FRIDGE

	QUANTITY	CALS	KJ
Pumpkin with Chunky Basil Pesto	20g	62	260
Triple Dip			
Basil Pesto, Cream Cheese & Sundried Tomato	20g	72	303
Rhubarb, Cream Cheese & Cashew & Pistachio Pesto	20g	65	275
Sweet Chilli, Cream Cheese & Coriander Pesto	20g	77	324
MASTER CHEF			
Pâté			
Chicken & Cognac	10g	29	124
Cracked Pepper	10g	27	114
Smoked Salmon	10g	27	114
MEDITERRANEAN			
Chunky Dip, Feta & Spinach	100g	499	2090
Hummus			
Roasted Garlic	100g	216	905
Sundried Tomato	100g	213	895
Layered Dip			
Pansotti	100g	346	1450
Margherita	100g	375	1570
Messicamo	100g	358	1500
Pesto			
Basil	100g	547	2290
Basil & Tomato	100g	420	1760
Feta & Spinach with Cashew & Parmesan	100g	500	2100
Roasted Capsicum	100g	461	1930
Sundried Tomato	100g	564	2360
OLD EL PASO			
Salsa			
Chunky Capsicum, Mild	100g	37	155
Chunky Chargrilled	100g	40	168
Chunky Tomato, Medium	100g	34	144
Chunky Tomato, Hot	100g	31	133
Roasted Capsicum	100g	74	310

	QUANTITY	CALS	KJ
Spicy Bean, Medium	100g	80	338
Thick 'n Chunky, Medium	100g	24	103
Thick 'n Chunky, Mild	100g	31	133

PAMS

Dip

Original Hummus	20g	44	188
Roasted Capsicum	20g	43	184
Spinach & Feta	20g	39	164
Sundried Tomato & Garlic	20g	44	185
Fresh Basil Pesto	20g	103	433

Pâté

Chicken & Port	12g	37	155
Farmhouse	12g	29	125

SIGNATURE RANGE

Basil & Pinenut Pesto	100g	371	1550
Guacamole	100g	114	480

Hummus

Moroccan Spice & Garlic	100g	172	720
Original	100g	179	750
Pumpkin & Kumara	100g	146	615
Roasted Capsicum	100g	168	705
Sundried Tomato	100g	176	740

Pâté

Cracked Pepper	100g	313	1310
Farmhouse	100g	341	1010

Salsa

Hot	100g	86	360
Medium	100g	86	360
Mild	100g	86	360

TARARUA

Dip

Creamy Onion	100g	167	700
Gherkin Relish	100g	174	730
Roasted Garlic & Onion	100g	169	710
Sour Cream & Chives	100g	167	700

FROM THE FRIDGE

	QUANTITY	CALS	KJ
Sweet Chilli	100g	169	710
THE GOOD TASTE COMPANY			
Black Label			
Capsicum, Coriander & Traditional Hummus	100g	193	810
Kiwi Onion Dip	100g	286	1200
Nacho Cheese & Salsa	100g	265	1110
Sundried Tomato, Traditional & Basil Hummus	100g	199	835
Sweet Chilli & Cream Cheese	100g	250	1050
Dip			
Cucumber & Mint Yoghurt	100g	105	440
Garlic & Onion	100g	361	1510
Garlic Lovers	100g	580	2430
Spinach & Ricotta	100g	261	1090
Double-Ups			
Basil Pesto Hummus with a Burst of Pesto	100g	234	980
Sundried Tomato Hummus with a Burst of Pesto	100g	211	885
Hummus			
Babaganoush	100g	223	935
Feta & Spinach	100g	181	759
Garlic Lovers	100g	215	900
Original	100g	192	805
Pumpkin & Kumara	100g	232	970
Sundried Tomato	100g	243	1020
Tomato & Capsicum	100g	223	935
Salsa, Tomato, Capsicum & Chilli	100g	140	585
SWISS DELI			
Liver Pâté, Coarse	100g	300	1259
Liver Pâté, Fine	100g	300	1259
TURKISH KITCHEN			
Dip			
Garlic & Cucumber	100g	109	458
Kumara & Lentil	100g	117	490

	QUANTITY	CALS	KJ
Spinach & Feta	100g	221	925
Yoghurt with Cucumber	100g	109	458
Flavour It Dips			
Smoked Salmon & Dill	100g	289	1210
Spinach & Basil	100g	585	2450
Hummus			
Manuka Smoked	100g	169	711
Traditional	100g	169	711

Pies & Pizza

BIG BEN

Pies			
Chicken & Gravy	each	335	1400
Mince	each	428	1790
Mince & Cheese	each	428	1790
Mince & Double Cheese	each	558	2330
Smokey Bacon & Egg	each	385	1610
Steak	each	419	1750
Steak & Cheese	each	440	1840

HOMEBRAND

Hawaiian	100g	258	1080
Supreme	100g	258	1080

IRVINES

700g Pies			
Cottage	100g	203	850
Mince	100g	227	950
Mince & Cheese	100g	239	1000
Party Pies			
Mince	each	157	660
Mince & Cheese	each	156	670
Pie Time			
Bacon & Egg	each	427	1790
Chicken & Vegetable	each	399	1670
Mince	each	430	1800
Mince & Cheese	each	463	1940
Potato Top	each	346	1450

FROM THE FRIDGE

	QUANTITY	CALS	KJ
Steak & Cheese	each	399	1670
Savouries			
Bacon & Egg	100g	157	660
Mince	100g	157	660
LA BAGUETTE			
Quiche			
Bacon & Egg Rounz	100g	262	1100
Bacon & Mozzarella	100g	238	996
Egg	100g	233	978
Spinach & Feta	100g	239	1000
LEANING TOWER			
Pizza Bases	100g	239	1000
Pizza Pronto			
BBQ Chicken	100g	258	1080
Hawaiian	100g	246	1030
Meat Lovers	100g	255	1070
Ultra Thin			
Angus Beef	100g	233	927
Moroccan Lamb	100g	222	927
MCCAIN			
Family Pizzas			
Ham & Pineapple	100g	230	963
Meat Lovers	100g	226	945
Supreme	100g	228	985
Pizza Singles, Ham & Pineapple	100g	223	932
Pizza Subs			
Ham & Pineapple	100g	223	932
Meat Lovers	100g	249	1040
MOMMAS			
Panini, Ham & Cheese	100g	219	919
Pizza			
Ham & Pineapple	100g	274	920
Meat Lovers	100g	301	1010
Rising Crush, Mexican	100g	197	828
Smoked Chicken	100g	362	985

	QUANTITY	CALS	KJ
Supreme	100g	288	970
Vegetable, Thin Crust Pizza	100g	207	870
PAMS, Handmade Pizza Base	100g	262	1100
PONSONBY PIES			
Pies			
Bacon & Egg	each	735	3078
Chicken & Kumara	each	678	2839
Chicken & Vegetable	each	661	2766
Cottage	each	505	2115
Mince	each	612	2568
Mince & Cheese	each	690	2888
Minted Lamb	each	590	2469
Pepper Steak	each	623	2608
Smoked Fish	each	616	2578
Spicy Vegetable	each	551	2307
Steak	each	606	2538
Steak & Cheese	each	707	2961
Steak & Mushroom	each	576	2413
PUREBREAD, Corn & Seed Pizza Bases	100g	231	969
ROMANO'S			
Pizza Bases			
Crispy, Tomato & Herb, Large	100g	146	1390
Honey & Olive Oil, Large	100g	93	1200
Honey & Olive Oil, Medium	100g	298	1250
Pizzas			
BBQ Meatlovers	100g	255	1070
Ham & Pineapple	100g	293	1230
Supreme	100g	298	1250
THE CHICAGO PIZZA COMPANY			
Pizza			
Ham & Pineapple	100g	233	972
Meat Lovers	100g	239	1000
Vegetarian			
BEAN SUPREME			
Felafel Burgers	100g	242	1013

FROM THE FRIDGE

	QUANTITY	CALS	KJ
Felafel Koftas	100g	242	1013
Gourmet Burgers	90g	239	1002
Lentil Koftas	100g	253	1060
Marinated Tofu			
Ginger & Honey	100g	178	749
Hoisin & Sesame	100g	165	694
Mushroom Burgers	75g	150	629
Tofu			
Firm Style	100g	105	442
Organic	100g	128	537
Vegetarian Meatballs	100g	132	554
Vegetarian Mince in Bolognese Sauce	100g	81	341
Vegetarian Sausages			
Roast Red Onion & Parmesan	2 sausages	200	838
Roasted Garlic	2 sausages	171	719
Rosemary, Sage & Parsley	2 sausages	201	843
Sundried Tomatoes & Kalamata Olive	2 sausages	194	814
FRY'S			
Traditional Burgers	each	119	501
Sausages, Banger-style Traditional	each	77	325
Schnitzel	100g	209	880
OLIVE GROVE			
Gluten Free Falafel Mix	100g	190	798
Traditional Falafel Mix	100g	100	421
SANITARIUM			
Vegie Delights			
Curried Sausages	100g	218	915
Hot Dogs	100g	201	840
Rashers	100g	234	980
Rosemary, Sage & Parsley Sausages	100g	158	662
Tender Fillets	100g	151	630
Vegie Sausages	100g	218	911
THE SOY WORKS, Vegetarian Sausages, Cajun	100g	151	635

	QUANTITY	CALS	KJ

Fruit (Fresh & Dried)

	QUANTITY	CALS	KJ
Apple			
dried	100g	243	1016
fresh	1 medium	95	396
Apricot			
dried	½	8	35
fresh	1 medium	17	70
Avocado	100g	160	669
Banana			
chips	100g	519	2169
fresh	1 medium	105	439
Blackberries	100g	43	180
Blackcurrants	100g	231	966
Blueberries	100g	57	238
Boysenberries	100g	50	209
Breadfruit	100g	103	431
Cantaloupe Melon	100g	34	142
Cherries, fresh	100g	63	263
Maraschino	100g	165	690
Coconut			
dried	100g	474	1981
fresh	1 cup	283	1183
Cranberries	100g	323	1350
Currants			
dried	100g	283	1183
fresh	100g	63	263
Custard Apple	100g	101	422
Dates, *dried*	100g	300	1255
Feijoa	1 medium	25	102
Figs			
dried	100g	286	1195
fresh	1 medium	37	155
Grapefruit	1 medium	41	171

FRUIT (FRESH & DRIED)

	QUANTITY	CALS	KJ
Grapes	100g	69	288
Green Gooseberries	100g	44	184
Guava	100g	68	284
Kiwifruit	1 medium	49	202
Kumquats	100g	71	297
Lemon	1 medium	17	70
Lime	1 medium	20	84
Loganberries	100g	55	230
Loquats	1 medium	8	31
Lychees	1 medium	6	25
Mandarin	1 medium	47	195
Mango			
dried	100g	75	313
fresh	100g	65	272
Melon			
dried	100g	17	71
fresh	100g	34	142
Mulberries	100g	43	180
Nashi Pear	1 medium	51	214
Nectarine	1 medium	62	261
Olives (Green/Black)	100g	233	973
Orange	1 medium	62	257
Papaya/Pawpaw	100g	39	163
Passionfruit	1 medium	17	73
Peach			
dried	½	31	130
fresh	1 medium	38	160
Pear			
dried	½	47	197
fresh	1 medium	96	402
Persimmon	1 medium	118	492
Pineapple			
dried	2 rings	130	543
fresh	thick slice	42	176
Plum	each	30	127

	QUANTITY	CALS	KJ
Pomegranate	1 medium	234	978
Prunes, *dried*	1 medium	20	84
Quince	1 medium	52	219
Raisins	100g	299	1250
Raspberries	100g	52	217
Rhubarb, no sugar, *stewed*	100g	21	88
Rock Melon	100g	30	126
Strawberries	100g	32	134
Sultanas	100g	320	1337
Tamarillo	1 medium	22	90
Tangelo	1 medium	47	196
Tangerine	1 medium	47	195
Tomato			
Cherry	1 medium	3	13
Regular	1 medium	22	93
Ugli Fruit	100g	28	118
Watermelon	100g	30	125
White Currants	100g	56	234

Meat

BEEF			
Corned Brisket	280g	917	3850
Corned Silverside	100g	326	1360
Dripping	1 tbsp	127	532
Fresh	280g	717	3010
Hamburger Patties	100g	262	1100
Kidney	100g	172	718
Liver, in flour, lean	100g	175	732
Luncheon Sausage	100g	321	1343
Meatballs	3 small	254	1068
Mince	100g	213	893
Nuggets	25g	63	262
Olives, no gravy	2	349	1466
Ox			

MEAT

	QUANTITY	CALS	KJ
Kidney	280g	240	1010
Tail	280g	260	1090
Tail, braised	per serve	309	1299
Rissoles	100g	121	507
Roast, lean	100g	326	1365
Rump, *grilled*	100g	159	663
Salami, Pepperoni	100g	382	1600
Sausage			
Cabanossi	100g	218	913
Frankfurter	100g	330	1382
fried	100g	332	1391
Schnitzel, *crumbed*	100g	215	896
Scotch Fillet, *grilled*	100g	195	815
Steak			
Blade	100g	248	1040
Chuck	100g	268	1122
Diane	225g	592	2480
Eye Fillet	100g	178	745
Filet Mignon	100g	191	800
Porterhouse	100g	210	879
Ribeye	85g	165	691
Sirloin	100g	183	763
Skirt	100g	201	842
T-Bone	100g	125	523
Tongue, *boiled*	85g	241	1009
Topside Roast	100g	183	766
Tripe, *dressed*	100g	94	393
Veal, *roasted*	100g	230	961
GAME			
Hare	100g	124	520
Kangaroo	100g	98	410
Rabbit	100g	173	724
Venison			
fresh	100g	153	641
Hamburger Patties	100g	186	779

	QUANTITY	CALS	KJ
Wild Pig			
no fat	280g	742	3116
with fat	280g	991	4163
LAMB			
Brains	100g	145	607
Chop			
fried	100g	336	1408
grilled	100g	132	553
Cutlets, lean, *grilled*	85g	160	670
Forequarter	100g	131	548
Fry, *grilled*	280g	694	2907
Heart, whole, *roasted*	280g	669	2803
Kidney, *fried*	100g	155	648
Leg, lean, *roasted*	100g	191	800
Liver, in flour, *fried*	100g	232	968
Loin Chop	100g	208	869
Minced Casserole	1 cup	450	1890
Noisettes	100g	194	813
Rump Chop	100g	195	814
Shoulder, lean, *roasted*	100g	212	887
PORK			
Bacon, lean, *grilled*	100g	323	1350
Black Pudding	100g	127	532
Chops			
baked	each	284	1190
fried	each	374	1567
Crackling	100g	545	2283
Fillet	100g	210	879
Ham	100g	193	808
Liver, *grilled*	100g	165	691
Loin Medallion	each	135	565
Mince	100g	241	1009
Parma Ham	100g	229	959
Pâté	55g	185	775
Pickled Pork, *no fat*	100g	141	592

	QUANTITY	CALS	KJ
Prosciutto	50g	124	519
Roast			
no fat	85g	210	883
with fat	85g	320	1340
Sausage, *grilled*	each	81	339
Schnitzel, *fried*	100g	97	406
Shoulder, lean, *roasted*	85g	196	821
Spare Ribs on Bone	110g	320	1340
Steak			
Butterfly	175g	188	787
Ham, grilled	100g	105	440
Leg, grilled	280g	335	1403
VEAL			
Cutlet	125g	249	1043
Escalope, *fried*	85g	309	1294
Fillet, *roasted*	per slice	89	372
Schnitzel	350g	558	2338
Steak	per steak	274	1152

Nuts & Seeds

	QUANTITY	CALS	KJ
Almonds			
raw	100g	578	2418
roasted, salted	100g	600	2510
roasted, unsalted	100g	607	2540
Brazil Nuts	100g	677	2830
Cashews			
raw	100g	553	2314
roasted, salted	100g	581	2431
roasted, unsalted	100g	580	2427
Chia Seeds	100g	520	2180
Chia Seeds, White	100g	480	2050
Flaxseed, whole	30g	160	670
LSA	30g	167	700
Macadamia Nuts			

	QUANTITY	CALS	KJ
raw	100g	715	2990
roasted	100g	760	3180
Peanuts			
honey-roasted	100g	554	2320
raw	100g	570	2390
roasted, salted	100g	623	2610
roasted, unsalted	100g	587	2456
Pecans	100g	695	2910
Pine Nuts	100g	603	2520
Pistachios			
raw	100g	557	2330
roasted, salted	100g	585	2450
Pumpkin Seeds, *raw*	100g	566	2370
Sancha Inch Seeds	40g	243	1020
Sesame Seeds, *hulled*	100g	630	2640
Sesame Seeds, *unhulled*	100g	570	2400
Sunflower Seeds	100g	605	2530
Walnuts	100g	699	2930

Pasta, Grains & Rice
(prepared as directed, unless stated otherwise)

Dried Pasta			
BARILLA			
Integrate Pasta, all shapes	100g	350	1482
Pasta, all shapes	100g	361	1511
BLACKWOOD			
Hello Kitty Pasta	100g	178	745
BUDGET			
Instant Noodles			
Beef	100g	95	398
Chicken	100g	93	393
Chicken & Corn	100g	95	400
Oriental	100g	89	374
Pasta, all shapes	125g	360	1510

PASTA, GRAINS & RICE

	QUANTITY	CALS	KJ
CONTINENTAL			
Pasta & Sauce, unprepared			
Alfredo	per serve	125	523
Chicken Curry	per serve	161	673
Creamy Bacon Carbonara	per serve	161	673
Creamy Bacon Carbonara, Light	per serve	104	437
Creamy Mushroom & Bacon	per serve	122	513
Four Cheeses	per serve	138	577
Macaroni Cheese	per serve	139	580
Sour Cream & Chives	per serve	164	687
DIAMOND, prepared			
Boxed Lasagne Sheets	50g	176	740
Dino & Teddy Bear Shapes	140g	201	842
Dry Pasta, all shapes	140g	206	862
Gluten Free, all shapes	63g	221	925
Vege Spirals	140g	205	859
DIVELLA, Gluten Free Pasta, all shapes	100g	131	1510
FANTASTIC, prepared			
Bowl Noodles			
Beef	per serve	382	1600
Chicken	per serve	387	1620
Oriental	per serve	384	1610
Cup Noodles			
BBQ Beef	per serve	334	1399
Beef	per serve	326	1365
Chicken	per serve	331	1385
Chicken & Corn	per serve	326	1365
Chicken Chow Mein	per serve	377	1580
Crispy Bacon	per serve	327	1372
Oriental	per serve	329	1378
Gluten Free Cup Noodles			
Beef	per serve	35	149
Chicken	per serve	36	151
Instant Noodles, dry	per serve	477	1998
Long Life Noodles	per serve	356	1490

	QUANTITY	CALS	KJ
Mighty Meal Bowl Noodles			
Hearty Beef	per serve	466	1950
Hearty Chicken	per serve	475	1990
HEALTHERIES			
Simple, unprepared			
Spaghetti	100g	356	1510
Spirals	100g	356	1510
Rigatoni	100g	356	1510
HIGHMARK			
Crispy Noodles			
Cheese	100g	493	2060
Chicken	100g	486	2030
Oriental	100g	454	1896
Traditional	100g	495	2070
HOMEBRAND, Durum Wheat Pasta, all shapes	100g	361	1510
INDOMIE			
Instant Cup Noodles			
Mi Goreng	100g	212	890
Mi Goreng, BBQ Chicken	100g	210	880
Mi Goreng, Rendang	100g	321	1340
Mi Goreng, Satay	100g	207	870
Instant Noodles			
Mi Goreng	100g	240	1000
Mi Goreng, BBQ Chicken	100g	213	890
Mi Goreng, Satay	100g	230	940
KRAFT, EASY MAC	100g	132	555
MACRO, Organic Pasta, all shapes	100g	352	1470
MAGGI			
Snack on Pasta			
Alfredo	per serve	330	1390
Cheese & Bacon	per serve	330	1390
Creamy Cheese with Garlic	per serve	330	1390
Macaroni & Cheese	per serve	330	1390
Sour Cream & Chives	per serve	340	1340

PASTA, GRAINS & RICE

	QUANTITY	CALS	KJ
Three Cheeses	per serve	330	1380
Vegetable Rice Pasta, all shapes	100g	353	1492
ORGRAN			
Buckwheat Pasta Spirals	100g	352	1480
Corn & Vegetable Shells	100g	352	1417
Farm Animals, Rice & Corn Vegetable	100g	329	1390
Lasagne Mini Sheets	100g	327	1380
Multigrain with Quinoa Penne	100g	334	1410
Outback Animals Vegetable	100g	329	1390
Rice & Corn Penne	100g	348	1470
Rice & Millet Spirals	100g	351	1478
Vegetable Rice Penne	100g	353	1492
Vegetable Rice Spirals	100g	353	1492
PAMS			
Hokkien Noodles	100g	145	609
Udon Noodles	100g	145	609
SAN REMO			
Durum Wheat Pasta, all shapes	100g	363	1520
Egg Pasta, all shapes	100g	360	1512
Gluten Free Egg Pasta, all shapes	100g	353	1480
Vegeroni Pasta Shapes	100g	353	1480
Wholemeal Pasta	100g	354	1510
SELECT, Pasta, all shapes	100g	366	1530
SLENDIER			
Noodles	100g	8	34
Organic Fettucine	100g	8	34
Spaghetti	100g	10	41
TRIDENT			
2 Minute Noodles			
Hot & Spicy	100g	78	328
Laksa	100g	133	555
Tom Yum	100g	102	427
Chow Mein Soft Noodles	100g	169	706
Hokkien Noodles	100g	134	619
Noodle Man			

	QUANTITY	CALS	KJ
Beef	100g	295	494
Chicken	100g	295	413
Hot & Spicy	100g	108	453
Pad Thai Noodles	100g	132	554
Rice Stick Noodles	100g	53	220
Singapore Soft Noodles	100g	168	704
Udon Noodles, Original	100g	139	583
ZAFARELLI			
Durum Wheat, all shapes	100g	363	520
Lasagne	50g	181	759
Fresh Pasta & Rice			
DELMAINE			
Angel Hair	100g	152	640
Asparagus & Parmesan Ravioli	100g	182	765
Bacon & Roasted Capsicum Sachetti	100g	151	635
Beef & Tomato Ravioli	100g	147	619
Cheese & Spinach Ravioli	100g	162	680
Chicken & 3 Cheese Sacchetti	100g	153	642
Chicken & Basil Tortellini	100g	148	621
Chicken, Bacon & Mozzarella Ravioli	100g	140	589
Chicken, Cashew & Tarragon Tortellini	100g	153	644
Chicken Parmigiana Tortellini	100g	144	605
Egg Fettuccine	100g	152	640
Egg Lasagne	100g	152	640
Egg Tagliatelle	100g	152	640
Light Fettuccine	100g	138	579
Mista Fettuccine	100g	152	640
Mushroom & 3 Cheese Tortellini	100g	153	641
Potato Gnocchi	100g	206	866
Spaghetti	100g	152	640
Spiced Pumpkin Ravioli	100g	185	778
Spinach & 3 Cheese Ravioli	100g	187	785
DIAMOND, prepared			
Macaroni Cheese, Bacon	per serve	279	1170
Macaroni Cheese, Sour Cream & Chives	per serve	277	1160

PASTA, GRAINS & RICE

	QUANTITY	CALS	KJ
Rice Risotto			
BBQ Pork	per serve	260	1090
Chicken	per serve	258	1080
Chinese	per serve	262	1100
Indian	per serve	255	1070
Mushroom	per serve	255	1070
Roast Beef	per serve	258	1080
Roasted Vegetable	per serve	258	1080
Teriyaki	per serve	258	1080
Thai Green Curry	per serve	262	1100
PAMS			
Beef, Sundried Tomato & Parmesan Ravioli	100g	148	623
Chicken, Bacon & Mozzarella Tortellini	100g	144	605
Chicken & Herb Tortellini	100g	145	607
Egg Fettuccine	100g	157	661
Egg Spaghetti	100g	133	557
Lasagne Sheets	100g	253	1060
Pumpkin, Ricotta & Sage Ravioli	100g	159	666
Ricotta & Basil Ravioli	100g	165	693
Tricolour Fettuccine	100g	156	653
SAN REMO			
La Pasta			
Carbonara	per serve	113	474
Creamy Bacon	per serve	113	474
Single Snack			
Alfredo	per serve	344	1440
Carbonara	per serve	353	1480
Chicken Curry	per serve	305	1280
Chicken & Mushroom	per serve	339	1420
Creamy Bacon	per serve	353	1480
Creamy Cheese	per serve	344	1440
Macaroni Cheese	per serve	348	1460
Sour Cream & Chives	per serve	344	1440

	QUANTITY	CALS	KJ
SELECT			
Pasta & Sauce			
Alfredo	100g	116	487
Carbonara	100g	118	490
Cheese & Cracked Pepper	100g	98	408
Chicken Curry	100g	102	427
Macaroni Cheese	100g	150	625
SIGNATURE RANGE			
Beef & Tomato Ravioli	100g	182	764
Beef & Wine Tricolour Tortellini	100g	170	715
Chicken Tortellini	100g	169	710
Egg Fettuccine	100g	160	670
Egg Lasagne	100g	160	670
Spaghetti	100g	160	670
Spinach & Cheese Tortellini	100g	185	775
Tricolour Fettuccine	100g	193	810
Grains			
ANSLEY HARRIOTT, prepared excluding butter & oil			
Lemon, Mint & Parsley Couscous	130g	192	812
Spice Sensation Couscous	130g	178	753
Sundried Tomato & Garlic Couscous	130g	196	828
BLU GOURMET, Pearl Couscous	100g	369	1548
CERES ORGANICS, unprepared			
Amaranth	100g	371	1554
Ancient Grain Fusion	100g	367	1537
Black Quinoa	100g	388	1624
Buckwheat	100g	335	1402
Bulghur Wheat	100g	468	1960
Canihua, Baby Quinoa	100g	382	1600
Farro	100g	365	1530
Freekeh	100g	363	1520
Hulled Millet	100g	378	1582
Inca Red Quinoa	100g	388	1625
Kasha, Toasted Buckwheat	100g	342	1435

PASTA, GRAINS & RICE

	QUANTITY	CALS	KJ
Kibbled Wheat	100g	327	1372
Polenta, coarse	100g	362	1515
Polenta, quick cooking	100g	344	1440
Quinoa-Rice Blend	100g	367	159
Super Grain Mix	100g	368	1542
White Quinoa	100g	368	1540
Wholemeal Couscous	50g	188	787
Wholemeal Spelt Couscous	100g	352	1475
DIAMOND			
Chicken & Lemon Couscous, prepared	120g	277	1160
Moroccan Couscous, prepared	120g	278	1165
FREELICIOUS, Couscous	100g	359	150
SAN REMO, Couscous	100g	358	1500
SELECT			
Mediterranean Couscous	100g	126	525
Moroccan Couscous	100g	126	527
UNCLE BEN'S			
Mediterranean Couscous	per serve	211	884
Moroccan Couscous	per serve	218	914
Rice			
CERES ORGANICS, cooked, unless stated otherwise			
Arborio	100g	358	1499
Basmati, Brown	100g	370	1549
Basmati, White	100g	365	1528
Black	100g	362	1515
Brown Long Grain	100g	370	1549
Brown Short Grain	100g	362	1516
Jasmine Brown	100g	365	1528
Long Grain Medley	100g	366	1532
Red	100g	362	1515
Sushi	100g	358	1499
White Medium Grain Rice	100g	360	1507
HOMEBRAND			
Basmati	100g	137	578

	QUANTITY	CALS	KJ
Jasmine	100g	121	521
KING'S CHOICE			
Basmati, uncooked	100g	144	605
Ezi-cook Basmati	100g	111	468
Jasmine	100g	354	1480
Long Grain Rice	100g	351	1475
KOHINOOR			
Charminar Basmati, uncooked	100g	346	1447
Rice Treat			
Butter Chicken	100g	233	961
Chinese Fried Rice	100g	200	836
Paneer Tikka Biryani	100g	210	879
Tikka Masala Rice	100g	229	961
PAMS			
Basmati, uncooked	100g	363	1520
Jasmine, uncooked	100g	348	1460
Long Grain Rice, uncooked	100g	347	1456
Parboiled Rice, uncooked	100g	352	1473
SUNRICE			
90 Seconds, precooked			
Fragrant Jasmine Rice	100g	200	839
Indian Aromatic Brown Basmati	100g	151	633
Medium Grain Brown Rice	100g	187	781
Oriental Style Egg Fried Rice	100g	144	604
Stir Fry Brown Rice	100g	189	790
Arborio, uncooked	100g	352	1470
Basmati, uncooked	100g	359	1500
Brown Rice, uncooked	100g	356	1490
Jasmine, uncooked	100g	356	1490
Long Grain White, uncooked	100g	354	1480
Medium Grain Australian Calrose Rice, uncooked	100g	356	1490
Sushi Rice, uncooked	100g	352	1470
UNCLE BEN'S			
Brown Rice	100g	153	644

PASTA, GRAINS & RICE/POTATO CHIPS & SNACKS

	QUANTITY	CALS	KJ
Express			
Chinese	100g	195	659
Savoury Chicken	100g	159	666
Long Grain White	100g	344	1462
Special Rice			
Egg Fried	per serve	205	866
Chinese Style	per serve	208	875
Golden Vegetables	per serve	191	808
Mexican Style	per serve	195	823
Mushroom	per serve	196	829
Special Fried	per serve	196	286
Thai Sweet Chilli	per serve	178	754
Vegetable Pilau	per serve	209	884

Potato Chips & Snacks

180 DEGREES

Crispy Snacks, Larosh			
Black & White Sesame Seed	100g	430	800
Garlic & Linseed	100g	415	1740
Sea Salt & Olive Oil	100g	413	1730
ABE'S BAGEL BAKERY			
Bagel Crisps			
Caramelised Onion & Balsamic Vinegar	25g	112	469
Marlborough Sea Salt	25g	108	455
Natural	25g	111	464
Roasted Garlic	25g	110	462
Sour Cream & Chives	25g	116	486
Wood-fired BBQ	25g	108	455
Kids Bites			
BBQ	15g	62	260
Pizza	15g	62	260
ACT II			
Popcorn, prepared			
Butter	100g	470	1967

	QUANTITY	CALS	KJ
Butter Lovers	100g	526	2202
Kettle Corn	100g	515	2156
Light Butter	100g	507	2121
Salted	100g	507	2121
BLUEBIRD			
Burger Rings	100g	547	2290
Cheezels	100g	544	2280
Copper Kettle			
BBQ	100g	492	2060
Cheddar & Red Onion Vintage	100g	494	2070
Sea Salt	100g	499	2090
Sea Salt & Vinegar	100g	487	2040
Delisio			
Caramelised Onion & Balsamic Vinegar	100g	518	2170
Greek Tzatziki	100g	501	2100
Sea Salt	100g	535	2240
Sweet Chilli Relish	100g	504	2110
Disco's, Tangy Tomato	100g	544	2280
Grain Waves			
Golden Cheddar	100g	499	2090
Honey & Mustard	100g	506	2120
Salsa	100g	504	2110
Sour Cream & Chives	100g	499	2090
Kiwi As – Classic Kiwi Onion	100g	513	2150
Light Plus			
Sea Salt	100g	492	2060
Smoke House Sweet Chilli	100g	513	2150
Sour Cream & Chives	100g	480	2010
MAXX			
Crushed Salt & Vinegar	100g	506	2120
Hot & Spicy Chicken Wings	100g	513	2150
Ultimate BBQ Ribs	100g	516	2160
Originals			
Chicken	100g	523	2190
Green Onion	100g	525	2200

POTATO CHIPS & SNACKS

	QUANTITY	CALS	KJ
Ready Salted	100g	537	2250
Salt & Vinegar	100g	521	2180
Sour Cream & Chives	100g	525	2200
Rashuns	100g	542	2270
Thick Cut Chips			
Crispy Bacon	100g	511	2140
Ready Salted	100g	523	2190
Sour Cream & Chives	100g	506	2120
Thin Cut			
Chicken	100g	525	2200
Ready Salted	100g	538	2250
Salt & Vinegar	100g	521	2180
Twisties	100g	509	2130
Zigzags, Wicked Cheddar	100g	513	2150
DORITOS			
Cheese Supreme	100g	518	2170
Flamegrilled BBQ	100g	506	2120
Nacho Cheese	100g	516	2160
Salsa	100g	513	2150
Salted Original	100g	504	2110
Thai Sweet Chilli	100g	511	2140
ETA			
Good Bites			
BBQ	12g	52	220
Cheddar Cheese	12g	51	214
Sour Cream & Chives	12g	52	220
Kettles			
BBQ	40g	203	850
Honey Soy Chicken	40g	200	840
Ready Salted	40g	205	860
Roast Lamb & Mint	40g	205	860
Salt & Vinegar	40g	200	840
Spare Ribs	40g	200	840
Kettles, Krinkle Cut			
Black Pepper & Salt	40g	212	888

	QUANTITY	CALS	KJ
Extreme Salt & Vinegar	40g	210	882
Rack of Ribs	40g	211	883
Sancho Corn Chips			
Cheesey Cheese	50g	248	1040
Nacho Cheese	50g	250	1050
Salsa	50g	243	1020
SKOF			
BBQ Tripods	35g	200	840
Cheese & Bacon Sonics	35g	195	820
Cheese & Onion Munchos	30g	145	610
Cheese Balls	40g	215	900
Cheese Burgers	40g	219	920
Chicken Tripods	35g	203	850
Fiery Ranch Corn Chips	45g	224	940
Salt & Vinegar Tripods	35g	188	790
Spicy Tomato Munchos	30g	141	590
Tasty Cheese Corn Chips	45g	224	940
Tasty Cheese Tripods	35g	207	870
Solay			
Sea Salt	35g	185	770
Sea Salt & Vinegar	35g	186	780
Sour Cream & Chives	35g	184	760
SPUDS			
Ripple Cut, Chicken	40g	207	870
Ripple Cut, Ready Salted	40g	210	880
Ripple Cut, Salt & Vinegar	40g	205	860
Ripple Cut, Sour Cream & Chives	40g	207	870
Ripple Cut, Spring Onion	40g	205	860
Ripple Cut, The Works	40g	207	870
Thick Cut, Ready Salted	40g	210	880
Thick Cut, Sour Cream & Onion	40g	210	880
Thin Cut, Chicken	40g	205	860
Thin Cut, Ready Salted	40g	207	870
Thin Cut, Salt & Vinegar	40g	203	850

POTATO CHIPS & SNACKS

	QUANTITY	CALS	KJ
UpperCuts			
Chargrilled Chicken & Herb Delicut	40g	205	860
Feta & Garlic, Corn Tapas	45g	227	950
Garlic & Sesame Crostini	100g	394	1650
Sea Salt, Corn Tapas	45g	227	950
Sea Salt & Balsamic Vinegar Delicut	40g	205	860
Sea Salt Delicut	40g	210	880
Sweet Chilli Relish Delicut	40g	205	860
Vintage Cheddar, Corn Tapas	45g	227	950
GARDEN OF EATIN'			
Corn Chips			
Blue	28g	140	585
Chilli & Lime	28g	140	585
Mini Yellow Rounds	28g	140	585
Nacho Cheese	28g	140	585
Red	28g	140	585
Sesame Blue	28g	150	627
HEALTHERIES			
Air Popped Potato Bites			
Sea Salt & Balsamic Vinegar	20g	82	343
Sour Cream & Chives	20g	82	344
Corn Pop Bites			
Lightly Buttered	20g	84	350
Sweet & Salty	20g	84	351
Corn Tubes			
Cheese	15g	56	233
Chicken	15g	55	229
Potato Pop Bites			
Roast Chicken & Herbs	20g	83	346
Sea Salt & Balsamic Vinegar	20g	82	343
Sour Cream & Chives	20g	82	344
Potato Stix			
Chicken	20g	86	358
Roast Potato	20g	89	362
Salt 'n Vinegar	20g	86	358

	QUANTITY	CALS	KJ
Rice Rounds			
BBQ	25g	83	345
Cheese & Bacon	25g	98	411
Original	25g	98	408
Rice Wheels			
Burger	18g	78	329
Cheese	18g	78	329
Sour Cream & Chives	18g	77	321
HOMEBRAND			
Cassava Vegetable Crisps			
BBQ	100g	504	2110
Original	100g	530	2220
Sour Cream & Chives	100g	504	2110
Thai Sweet Chilli	100g	497	2080
KENNY'S			
Kumara Chips			
Natural	40g	192	804
Salt & Pepper	40g	190	796
Sour Cream & Chives	40g	190	796
MEXICANO			
Corn Chips			
Cheese	30g	143	600
Jalapeno	30g	142	598
Natural	30g	146	611
PAMS			
Cassava Vegetable Crisps			
BBQ	100g	504	2110
Original	100g	525	2200
Sour Cream & Chives	100g	504	2110
Cheesy Aliens	100g	210	2380
Cheesy Twists	100g	234	2460
Classic			
Cheese & Onion	100g	568	2150
Chicken	100g	521	2180
Green Onion	100g	511	2140

POTATO CHIPS & SNACKS

	QUANTITY	CALS	KJ
Ready Salted	100g	550	2220
Salt & Vinegar	100g	513	2150
Sour Cream & Chives	100g	518	2170
Corn Chips			
BBQ Classic	100g	470	1970
Chilli & Lime	100g	473	1980
Double Cheese	100g	475	1990
Salsa Party	100g	470	1970
Kettle Fried Chips			
BBQ	100g	516	2160
Ready Salted	100g	501	2100
Salt & Vinegar	100g	506	2120
Microwave Popcorn			
Butter	100g	521	2180
Extra Butter	100g	547	2290
Lite Butter	100g	411	1720
Kettle	100g	501	2100
Natural	100g	521	2180
Spicy Bhuja Mix	100g	504	2110
POP'N'GOOD			
Popcorn			
Bacon & Cheese	12g	59	251
Butter Max	100g	532	2730
Caramel	100g	425	1780
Frutti	100g	432	1810
Light & Buttery	12g	55	232
Sensations, Caramel & Cashew	100g	473	1980
Sensations, Chocolate & Caramel	100g	518	2170
Sensations, Organic Manuka Honey	100g	401	1680
Sweet & Salty	100g	490	2051
PRINGLES			
Honey Mustard	28g	150	627
Original	28g	150	627
Salt & Vinegar	28g	150	627
Sour Cream & Onion	28g	150	627

	QUANTITY	CALS	KJ
RED ROCK DELI			
Lime & Black Pepper	100g	494	2070
Honey Soy Chicken	100g	492	2060
Sea Salt	100g	487	2040
Sweet Chilli	100g	489	2050
SIGNATURE RANGE			
Crinkle Cuts			
Chicken	100g	519	2170
Green Onion	100g	512	2140
Ready Salted	100g	526	2200
Salt & Vinegar	100g	514	2150
Sour Cream & Chives	100g	519	2170
Kettles			
Barbecue	100g	507	212
Ready Salted	100g	517	2160
Tortilla Chips			
Chilli & Lime	100g	492	2060
Double Cheese	100g	499	2090
Tangy Salsa	100g	497	2080
WELLABY'S			
Kalamata Olive, Hummus Chips	30g	126	527
Rosemary, Lentil Chips	30g	120	502
WEIGHT WATCHERS			
Crinkle Crisps			
Cheese & Onion	100g	411	1720
Potato Bakes, Sour Cream & Chives	100g	417	1745
Roast Chicken	100g	401	1680

Poultry

	QUANTITY	CALS	KJ
CHICKEN			
Breast, no skin	100g	165	690
Cordon Bleu	100g	197	824
Drumstick			
fried	100g	222	929

	QUANTITY	CALS	KJ
grilled	100g	167	697
roasted	100g	216	903
Finger, *crumbed*	each	100	418
Giblets	50g	139	579
Kiev	100g	271	1134
Liver Pâté	100g	201	840
Livers, *pan-fried*	100g	172	719
Nuggets	100g	167	699
Pie	100g	223	932
Roast, no skin	100g	165	690
Smoked, no skin	100g	89	373
DUCK			
Roast			
no skin	100g	189	788
with skin	100g	337	1409
GOOSE, Roast, no skin	100g	238	995
MUTTON BIRD, Pieces	100g	208	871
TURKEY			
Pieces	280g	298	1250
Roast, no skin	280g	398	1670

Ready Meals

PITANGO			
Curry			
Free Range Butter Chicken	200g	238	999
Free Range Thai Green Chicken	200g	188	788
Free Range Thai Red Chicken	200g	189	793
Kids Free Range Very Mild Chicken	200g	83	347
Organic Vegetable Korma	200g	106	447
Pasta			
Kids Macaroni Cheese	100g	150	631
Kids Organic Spaghetti Bolognese	100g	98	411
Macaroni & Cheese	400g	545	2283

	QUANTITY	CALS	KJ
Organic Penne with Tomato & Feta Sauce	400g	262	1100
Penne with Creamy Chicken & Herb Sauce	400g	628	2631
Penne with Creamy Portobello Mushroom Sauce	400g	135	568
Risotto			
Kids Salmon	100g	126	530
Organic Chicken & Garlic	250g	305	1277
Organic Pumpkin, Leek & Spinach	250g	218	915
Organic Tomato, Feta & Basil	250g	235	985
Salmon, Dill & Pumpkin	250g	202	847
SEALORD			
Heat & Eat			
Fish Pie with Tuna	100g	113	474
Green Curry with Tuna	100g	142	595
Italian Pasta & Tuna	100g	106	445
Red Curry with Tuna	100g	120	500
Satay Rice & Tuna	100g	183	769
Teriyaki Rice & Chicken	100g	132	555
SUNRICE			
Hokkien Noodles			
Basil & Chilli Chicken	per serve	141	591
Beef & Oyster Sauce	per serve	135	569
Teriyaki Chicken	per serve	151	633
Rice			
Beef & Black Bean	per serve	120	506
Butter Chicken Curry	per serve	145	609
Chicken Korma	per serve	158	664
Chicken Satay Curry	per serve	167	700
Chicken Tikka Masala	per serve	137	577
Chilli Con Carne	per serve	113	475
Green Chicken Curry	per serve	142	598
Massaman Chicken Curry	per serve	152	640
Moroccan Beef	per serve	144	606

READY MEALS

	QUANTITY	CALS	KJ
Red Chicken Curry	per serve	144	605
Sweet & Sour Chicken	per serve	134	564
TASTY POT			
Meal For One			
5 Grain Superpot	100g	66	280
Chicken Tikka Masala	100g	190	377
Thai Green Curry	100g	70	293
THE KAWEKA FOOD COMPANY			
Apricot Chicken	per serve	415	1740
Beans, Bangers & Bacon	per serve	396	1660
Butter Chicken	per serve	547	2290
NZ Beef & Red Wine	per serve	322	1350
NZ Lamb Casserole	per serve	270	1130
Thai Chicken	per serve	442	1850
WATTIE'S			
Big Eat			
All Day Breakfast	100g	124	520
Butter Chicken	100g	88	370
Lamb Rogan Josh	100g	72	305
Ravioli Bolognese	100g	90	380
Spaghetti Bolognese	100g	88	370
Ready to Serve Tortellini			
Creamy Mushroom & Bacon	per serve	413	1730
Creamy Pumpkin & Roast Garlic	per serve	284	1190
Sundried Tomato & Bacon	per serve	284	1190
WEIGHT WATCHERS	per serve	293	1230
Beef Hot Pot	per serve	208	872
Butter Chicken	per serve	358	1500
Chilli Con Carne	per serve	336	1409
Spanish Chicken	per serve	313	1310
Sweet & Sour Chicken	per serve	322	1351
Thai Green Chicken	per serve	328	1375
WOKKA			
Noodles with Bacon, Garlic & Chives Sauce	per serve	329	1377

	QUANTITY	CALS	KJ
Noodles with Roasted Peanut & Honey Soy Sauce	per serve	424	1777
Noodles with Sweet Chilli Chicken Sauce	per serve	474	1982
Noodles with Thai Peanut Satay Sauce	per serve	424	1777

Sauces, Condiments & Gravies
(prepared as directed, unless stated otherwise)

Gravy			
BISTO			
Gravy Mix			
Light Brown	100mL	29	120
Rich Brown	100mL	26	110
Supreme	100mL	28	117
Instant Gravy			
Classic Chicken	100mL	42	174
Tasty Brown Onion	100mL	41	173
Traditional Roast Meat	100mL	41	171
Liquid Gravy			
Roast Chicken with Herbs	100mL	41	170
Traditional	100mL	40	169
CONTINENTAL			
Instant Gravy			
Brown Onion	60mL	27	114
Light Brown	60mL	35	147
Rich Brown	60mL	32	136
Roast Chicken	60mL	34	142
Roast Meat	60mL	29	120
HOMEBRAND, Traditional Gravy Mix	100mL	33	141
MAGGI			
Brown Onion	100mL	38	160
Chicken & Herb	100mL	35	150
Country Roast & Rosemary	100mL	43	180

SAUCES, CONDIMENTS & GRAVIES

	QUANTITY	CALS	KJ
Garden Mint	100mL	35	150
Light Brown	100mL	40	170
Pork	100mL	40	169
Rich Brown	100mL	40	170
Rich Dark	100mL	23	100
Rich Meat	100mL	33	140
Roast Chicken	100mL	38	160
Roast Meat	100mL	40	170
Sage & Onion	100mL	43	180
MCCORMICK			
Classic Onion & Mushroom Gravy	100mL	37	158
Roast Beef Gravy	100mL	28	119
ORGRAN, Gluten Free Gravy Mix	100g	326	1376
PAMS			
Brown Onion	100mL	38	161
Chicken	100mL	41	175
Light Brown	100mL	40	169
Rich Brown	100mL	39	167
Roast Meat	100mL	40	169
WEIGHT WATCHERS			
Brown Onion	100mL	26	112
Country Chicken	100mL	27	113
Sauces & Condiments			
ANATHOTH			
Chutney			
Apricot	100g	153	644
Beetroot	100g	152	638
Fruit	100g	184	771
Spicy Green Tomato	100g	116	488
Farmstyle Pickle	100g	103	435
Garden Chow Chow	100g	116	489
Sweet Chilli Relish	100g	179	749
Tomato Relish	100g	110	461
Zucchini Pickle	100g	114	480

	QUANTITY	CALS	KJ
BARKER'S			
Chutney			
Capsicum & Apricot	10g	11	47
New Zealand Green Tomato	10g	15	66
Peach & Mango	10g	16	70
Ploughman's	10g	17	75
Roasted Vegetable	10g	9	40
Spiced Eggplant	10g	19	82
Sundried Tomato & Olive	10g	15	64
Jelly			
Blackcurrant & Red Onion	10g	21	88
Cranberry	10g	18	78
Mint & Apple	10g	31	132
New Zealand Redcurrant	10g	29	124
Red Peppers & Chilli	10g	18	76
New Zealand Beetroot Relish	10g	10	46
New Zealand Onion Marmalade	10g	17	72
BOSS, Worcestershire Mild Sauce	12mL	10	43
BUDGET, Tomato Relish	100g	140	586
CEREBOS			
Chow Chow	100g	122	509
Chunky Chow Chow	100g	125	521
Home Style Pickle	100g	127	528
Piccalilli	100g	117	488
Relish			
Sweet Corn	100g	146	610
Tangy Tomato	100g	156	651
Tomato	100g	155	649
CONTINENTAL			
Chicken Tonight Recipe Sauces			
97% Fat Free Golden Honey Mustard	100g	71	300
97% Fat Free Sweet & Sour	100g	107	450
Golden Honey Mustard	100g	144	603
Indian Chicken Tonight Recipe Sauces			
97% Fat Free Butter Chicken	100g	73	307

SAUCES, CONDIMENTS & GRAVIES

	QUANTITY	CALS	KJ
Butter Chicken	100g	112	472
Creamy Tandoori	100g	90	380
Packet Sauce			
Cheese	60mL	51	213
Four Cheeses	60mL	36	152
Pepper	60mL	35	147
White	60mL	45	190
COTTERILL & ROUSE			
Beetroot Relish with Orange	100g	164	687
Chutney, Tamarillo	100g	93	392
Onion Marmalade Relish	100g	143	601
Ploughman's Pickle Chutney	100g	155	649
Roasted Tomato Relish	100g	100	422
DELMAINE			
Chutney			
Apple & Date	25g	35	148
Mango & Lime	25g	27	113
Piccalilli	25g	21	91
Plum & Coriander	25g	37	157
Red Onion & Jalapeno	25g	18	78
Jelly			
Mint	15g	37	155
Redcurrant	15g	38	161
Pasta Sauces			
Alfredo	80g	151	632
Alfredo with Basil	80g	140	586
Basillico	80g	59	248
Carbonara	80g	113	476
Cipriani	80g	114	478
Creamy Portabello	80g	97	409
Original Spicy Tomato	80g	27	115
Pomodora	80g	30	126
Spinach & Blue Cheese	80g	103	432
Tomato & Roasted Garlic	80g	44	187
White Wine & Bacon	80g	131	549

SAUCES, CONDIMENTS & GRAVIES

	QUANTITY	CALS	KJ
Sauce			
Cranberry, Orange & Port	15g	21	91
Plum	15g	28	119
Smoked Manuka BBQ	15g	21	91
Tomato Relish	25g	21	92
Tomato Sauce with Chili	15g	18	78
Traditional Apple	15g	12	53
Traditional Apricot	15g	22	96
Traditional Mint	15g	20	87
Traditional Tomato	15g	20	85
DOLMIO			
Lasagne			
Bechamel	100g	124	519
Extra Cheese	100g	119	498
Thick Tomato	100g	74	313
Pasta Bake			
Creamy Mushroom	100g	108	456
Creamy Sundried Tomato & Garlic	100g	87	367
Creamy Tomato & Mozzarella	100g	102	429
Three Cheese	100g	117	493
Tomato with Extra Cheese	100g	91	384
Tuna Bake	100g	120	506
Pasta Sauces			
Extra Bolognese	100g	57	240
Extra Farmhouse Vegetables	100g	53	224
Extra Four Cheese	100g	56	237
Extra Garden Vegetables	100g	51	215
Extra Garlic	100g	55	234
Extra Italian Herbs	100g	60	255
Extra Mushroom	100g	52	220
Extra Red Wine & Italian Herbs	100g	60	254
Extra Spicy Peppers	100g	55	234
Extra Tomato, Onion & Roast Garlic	100g	58	244
Extra Tomato, Onion & Roast Garlic Salt Reduced	100g	56	237

SAUCES, CONDIMENTS & GRAVIES

	QUANTITY	CALS	KJ
Traditional Basil	100g	62	263
Traditional Classic Tomato	100g	65	273
Traditional Classic Tomato, Salt Reduced	100g	62	262
FIVE BROTHERS			
Pasta Sauce			
Alfredo	100g	120	502
Bolognese	100g	52	218
Boscaiola	100g	111	465
Carbonara	100g	115	481
Five Cheese	100g	58	241
Grilled Summer Vegetable	100g	52	91
Oven Roasted Garlic & Onion	100g	48	200
Oven Roasted Garlic with Wine	100g	50	212
Portobello Mushroom & Garlic	100g	45	188
Summer Tomato & Basil	100g	43	183
GOLDEN SUN			
Sweet Thai Chilli Sauce	100mL	236	988
Sweet Thai Chilli Sauce with Ginger	100mL	232	974
GREGG'S			
Sauce			
Classic BBQ	100mL	182	760
Lite Tomato	100mL	90	375
Mint	100mL	132	550
Rich Red Tomato	100mL	145	605
Rich Steak	100mL	195	813
Smoked Hickory	100mL	175	730
Sweet Chilli	100mL	191	800
HEINZ			
Sauce			
Organic Tomato Ketchup	100mL	126	530
Tomato Ketchup	100mL	129	540
Seriously Good Pasta Sauce			
Four Cheeses	100g	96	405
Tomato & Roasted Garlic	100g	62	260
Tomato & Sweet Basil	100g	64	270

	QUANTITY	CALS	KJ
HIGHMARK SAUCE			
Low Salt	100mL	47	200
Premium Dark	100mL	39	167
Premium Golden	100mL	23	99
Reduced Salt	100mL	63	264
Soy Sauce, Organic	100mL	47	199
Tamari	100mL	47	199
HOMEBRAND			
HP Sauce			
BBQ	15g	20	84
Original	15g	18	78
Sauce			
BBQ	100mL	184	770
Tomato	100mL	89	370
Taco	100mL	50	213
JOK'N'AL			
Tomato Ketchup	30g	15	64
Tomato Relish	30g	16	69
KAITAIA FIRE			
Pepper Sauce, Chilli	100g	245	1027
Waha Wera, Pepper Sauce	100g	132	556
KAN TONG			
Butter Chicken	100g	133	556
Chinese Barbeque	100g	88	370
Inspirations			
Honey, Soy & Garlic	80g	65	274
Teriyaki Sesame	80g	103	435
Peanut Satay	100g	124	519
Pineapple Sweet & Sour	100g	103	434
Sweet & Sour	100g	97	410
KATO			
Classic Hollandaise	100mL	658	2755
Lite Hollandaise	100mL	298	1250
Malabar Peppercorn Sauce	100mL	636	2665

SAUCES, CONDIMENTS & GRAVIES

	QUANTITY	CALS	KJ
KIKKOMAN			
Gluten Free Soy Sauce	100mL	101	422
Less Salt Soy Sauce	100mL	127	599
Soy Sauce	100mL	98	411
Tasman Soy Sauce	100mL	125	524
Teriyaki Marinade	100mL	117	490
LEGGO'S			
Pasta Bake			
Creamy Sundried Tomato & Garlic	100g	72	303
Creamy Tomato Mozzarella	100g	70	294
Tomato, Ricotta & Spinach	100g	84	355
Tuna Bake	100g	100	419
Pasta Sauce			
Bolognese	100g	76	318
Carbonara	100g	94	397
Mushroom Bolognese	100g	60	251
Red Wine Bolognese	100g	73	309
Pizza Sauce	100g	53	224
Stir-Through			
Ricotta, Spinach & Pecorino Cheese	100g	156	653
Sundried Tomato & Roasted Garlic	100g	123	517
Tomato Paste, No Added Salt	100g	65	275
Tomato Paste, Original	100g	68	287
LEA & PERRINS, Original Worcestershire Sauce	5mL	5	20
MAGGI			
Gluten Free			
Roast Chicken	100mL	43	180
Tasty Cheese	100mL	71	300
Instant Sauce Mixes			
Cheese	100mL	74	310
Cheese, Onion & Herb	100mL	74	310
Cracked Pepper	100mL	59	250
Creamy White	100mL	57	240
Hollandaise	100mL	126	530

	QUANTITY	CALS	KJ
Parsley	100mL	53	223
Tasty Cheese	100mL	71	300
MAILLE			
Aïoli	15g	93	390
Béarnaise	15g	95	390
Dijon	15g	15	65
Dijonnaise	15g	63	270
Hollandaise	15g	74	300
Tartare	15g	89	360
Wholegrain Mustard	15g	20	75
MAISON THERESE			
Relish			
Balsamic Onion	100g	100	421
Beetroot	100g	114	479
MASTERFOODS			
Marinades			
Red Wine & Garlic	37g	45	192
Satay	37g	62	236
Smokey BBQ	37g	50	213
Soy, Honey & Garlic	37g	57	239
Teriyaki	37g	66	278
Mint Jelly	37g	53	225
Mustard			
American	10g	11	49
Dijon	10g	12	54
Dijonnaise	10g	22	96
Honey	10g	15	66
Honey, Wholegrain	10g	20	86
Horseradish Cream	10g	18	76
Hot English	10g	6	68
Mild English	10g	10	46
Wholegrain	10g	12	53
Sauces			
BBQ	10mL	25	106
Honey Barbecue	15mL	30	126

SAUCES, CONDIMENTS & GRAVIES

	QUANTITY	CALS	KJ
Hot Chilli	10mL	9	40
Sweet & Sour	20g	28	119
Sweet Chilli	10mL	24	104
Tomato	15mL	21	88
Tomato & Sweet Chilli	15mL	37	155
Tomato Ketchup	15mL	20	87
Traditional Tartare	10g	61	258
MCILHENNY CO., Tabasco	5mL	3	11
MRS H.S. BALL'S			
Chutney			
Hot	100g	187	783
Original	100g	188	788
Peach	100g	183	787
NANDO'S			
Marinades			
Hot Peri-Peri Chicken	100mL	115	484
Lemon & Herb Chicken	100mL	99	414
Peri-Peri Chicken	100mL	61	244
Portuguese BBQ Chicken	100mL	90	380
Sauce			
Peri-Peri, Extra Hot	100mL	71	298
Peri-Peri, Hot	100mL	75	14
OCEAN SPRAY			
Jellied Cranberry Sauce	¼ cup	110	460
Whole Berry Cranberry Sauce	¼ cup	110	460
PAMS			
Chow Chow	100g	125	524
Lite Tomato Sauce	100mL	80	335
Packet Sauces			
Cheese	100mL	34	267
Parsley	100mL	75	314
Tasty Cheese	100mL	49	307
Piccalilli	100g	123	515
Sweet Fruit Chutney	100g	142	596
Sweet Mustard Pickle	100g	157	658

	QUANTITY	CALS	KJ
Tomato Relish	100g	142	597
Tomato Sauce	100mL	118	494
Worcestershire Sauce	100mL	79	334
PITANGO			
Cranberry Port & Orange	50g	46	194
Organic Apple	50g	32	135
SABATO			
Bruschetta Toppings			
Caper	28g	75	315
Olive	28g	77	323
Pepperoni	28g	49	206
Porcini	28g	86	354
Tomato	28g	86	360
Chutneys & Sauces			
Julie Le Clerc Arabian Date	15mL	52	216
Julie Le Clerc Balsamic Honey Mustard	15mL	40	169
Julie Le Clerc Beetroot Salsa	15mL	23	95
Julie Le Clerc Capsicum Chilli Jam	15mL	46	191
Julie Le Clerc Moroccan Chutney	15mL	33	139
Julie Le Clerc Smoked Paprika Tomato Sauce	15mL	20	82
Julie Le Clerc Spicy Harissa	15mL	18	74
Peter Gordon Chunky Fig, Walnut & Whiskey Chutney	15mL	38	160
Peter Gordon Famous Sweet Chilli Sauce	15mL	28	118
Peter Gordon Fiery Red Chilli Relish	15mL	36	150
Peter Gordon Moorish Moroccan Relish	15mL	25	104
Peter Gordon Sunny Avocado Oil & Pomegranate Molasses Dressing	15mL	86	359
Mayonnaise			
Egg	15g	107	447
Garlic Aioli	15g	106	445
Mustard Mayonnaise	15g	101	424
Tartare Mayonnaise	15g	90	376
Pasta Sauce			
Basil	100mL	71	298

SAUCES, CONDIMENTS & GRAVIES

	QUANTITY	CALS	KJ
Eggplant	100mL	76	219
Fungi Porcini	100mL	65	273
Peppers & Chilli	100mL	79	332
Puttanesca	100mL	89	376
Ricotta Forte	100mL	77	326
Rocket	100mL	107	449
Tomato Passata	100mL	32	136
Pesto & Pastes			
Pesto All'arrabbiata	18g	75	313
Pesto Alla Genovese	30g	258	1080
Pesto Sweet Peppers	18g	80	334
Porcini Crema	30g	54	226
Pronto Rosso	15g	72	300
Salsa Verde	30g	154	646
SELECT SAUCE			
Apple	100mL	50	208
Hoi Sin	100mL	329	1380
Hot Chilli	100mL	83	345
Oyster	100mL	164	689
Portuguese Chicken	100mL	106	444
Seafood	100mL	406	1700
Singapore Satay	100mL	157	661
Soy, Garlic & Honey	100mL	151	634
Sweet Chilli	100mL	210	882
Teriyaki	100mL	133	560
Thick Mint	100mL	158	665
Tomato	100mL	163	685
Worcestershire	100mL	85	355
SIGNATURE RANGE			
Chow Chow	100g	127	535
Mustard Pickle Relish	100g	88	371
Piccalilli	100g	125	525
Spiced Apricot Chutney	100g	153	643
Sweet Fruit Chutney	100g	158	665
Tangy Tomato Relish	100g	124	520

	QUANTITY	CALS	KJ
Tomato Relish	100g	127	532
TRIDENT			
Sweet Chilli Sauce	100mL	292	1220
Sweet Chilli Sauce, Hot	100mL	311	1300
Sweet Chilli Sauce with Ginger	100mL	313	1310
Sweet Chilli Sauce with Lime	100mL	311	1300
WATTIE'S			
Bit on the Side Sauces			
Absolute Apple	100g	148	205
Cracker Cranberry	100g	125	525
Java Satay	100g	179	750
Oriental Plum	100g	137	575
Spiced Apricot	100g	187	785
Sweet Chilli	100g	161	675
Teriyaki	100g	121	510
Curry Sauces			
Creamy Butter Chicken	100g	124	520
Creamy Satay	100g	139	585
Honey Soy & Ginger	100g	101	425
Korma	100g	88	370
European Creations Simmer Sauces			
Beef Bourguignon	100g	74	310
Stroganoff	100g	78	330
Indian Creations Curry Sauces			
Butter Chicken	100g	111	465
Korma	100g	94	395
Tikka Masala	100g	95	400
Italian Creations Pasta Sauces			
Carbonara	100g	84	355
Creamy Three Cheese	100g	96	405
Creamy Tomato & Parmesan	100g	84	355
Tomato & Basil Pesto	100g	65	275
Tomato & Roasted Garlic	100g	59	250
Tomato, Red Wine & Balsamic	100g	53	225
Just Add Simmer Sauces			

SAUCES, CONDIMENTS & GRAVIES

	QUANTITY	CALS	KJ
Butter Chicken	100g	89	375
Cottage Pie	100g	47	200
Country French Mince	100g	37	155
Curry Mince	100g	65	275
Devilled Sausages	100g	51	215
Hearty Savoury Mince	100g	43	180
Sweet & Sour Chicken	100g	101	425
Sweet Apricot Chicken	100g	72	305
Mexican Creations Simmer Sauce			
Burrito	100g	50	210
Chilli Con Carne	100g	57	240
Nachos	100g	53	225
Sauces			
BBQ	100g	117	490
Homestyle Tomato	100g	127	535
Ketchup	100g	114	480
Lite Tomato	100g	102	430
Steak	100g	144	605
Sweet & Sour	100g	126	530
Sweet Chilli	100g	157	660
Tomato	100g	136	570
Wok Creations Stir Fry Sauces			
Chinese BBQ	100g	131	550
Honey Soy	100g	163	685
Lemon, Ginger & Sesame	100g	141	590
Malaysian Peanut Satay	100g	182	765
Pad Thai	100g	144	605
Sweet & Sour	100g	130	545
Sweet Chilli & Lime	100g	191	800
Teriyaki	100g	172	720
WHITLOCK'S			
Caramelised Onion Chunky Relish	100g	163	681
Peach, Mango & Apricot Spiced Chutney	100g	146	609
Sauces			
Hot Mexican Chilli	100mL	184	770

	QUANTITY	CALS	KJ
Mint	100mL	120	500
Peanut Satay	100mL	240	1005
Smoky BBQ	100mL	197	825
Soy	100mL	53	220
Worcestershire	100mL	62	260

Snack Bars & Slices

ARTISSE, Organic Avibar Cocoa	each	92	384
BE NATURAL			
Nut Bars			
Apricot Almond	each	184	770
Macadamia Honey	each	253	1060
Nut Delight	each	212	890
Trail Bars			
Berry	each	109	460
Dark Chocolate	each	119	500
Honey Nut	each	114	480
Nut & Fruit	each	114	480
BROOKFARM Bar, Baked with Macadamias & Cranberries	each	156	654
CADBURY			
Brunch Bars			
Hazelnut	each	167	699
Mixed Berry	each	151	634
Peanut	each	179	749
Toasted Coconut	each	160	672
CARMAN'S			
Apricot & Almond Muesli Bar	each	200	838
Dark Choc, Blueberry Superfood Bar	each	166	693
Dark Choc, Cranberry & Almond Bar	each	163	683
Deluxe Gluten Free Muesli Bar	each	160	669
Fruit & Nut Muesli Bar	each	196	819
Fruit-Free Muesli Bar	each	201	842
Yoghurt, Apricot & Almond Bar	each	163	683

SNACK BARS & SLICES

	QUANTITY	CALS	KJ
CERES			
Raw Food Bars			
Apple Cinnamon	each	199	833
Apricot Almond	each	202	848
Cashew	each	217	910
Ginger	each	200	839
LSA	each	203	853
COOKIE TIME			
Bumper Bars			
Apricot Chocolate	each	347	1450
Banana Chocolate	each	350	1460
Raspberry White Chocolate	each	349	1460
Wildberry Chocolate	each	348	1460
One Square Meal, all flavours	each	347	1450
One Square Meal Bite, all flavours	each	173	725
FLEMINGS			
Chewy Muesli Bar			
Apricot Choc Chip	each	119	500
Choc Chip	each	119	500
Very Berry	each	119	500
Kiwi-Licious			
Hokey Pokey	each	113	476
Pineapple Chunks	each	113	473
Rocky Mallow	each	116	486
Snacker, Double Choc	each	88	370
HOMEBRAND			
Fruit Bars, all flavours	each	79	332
Muesli Bar, Strawberry Yoghurt	each	104	435
Oven Baked Fruit Bar			
Apple	each	120	503
Apple & Blueberry	each	121	507
KELLOGG'S			
LCMs			
Choc Chips	each	93	90
Kaleidos	each	90	380

	QUANTITY	CALS	KJ
Original	each	93	390
Nutri-Grain	each	124	520
Special K Chocolatey Bar, Caramel	each	88	370
Special K Chocolatey Bar, Raspberry	each	88	370
Split-Stix, Chocolatey	each	97	410
Split-Stix, Yoghurty	each	100	420
LEDA, Baked Fruit Filled Bars, all flavours	each	119	500
MOTHER EARTH			
Baked Oaty Singles			
Apricot Chocolate	each	159	668
Choc Chip	each	306	1283
Baked Oaty Slices			
Afghan	each	175	736
Almonds, Grains & Honey	each	181	760
Anzac	each	172	720
Apple Crumble	each	155	650
Apricot Chocolate	each	159	668
Choc Chip	each	175	733
Chocolate Orange	each	168	704
Raspberry & White Chocolate	each	169	708
Sticky Date Pudding	each	153	644
Sultana, Oat & Honey	each	155	652
Brekkie On The Go			
Apricot & Almond	each	181	761
Cashew & Cranberry	each	189	792
Hazelnut & Dark Chocolate	each	204	855
Fruit Sticks			
Apple	each	60	253
Apple & Peach	each	65	272
Apple & Raspberry	each	57	239
Apple & Strawberry	each	60	252
Apricot	each	60	253
Blueberry	each	61	257
Pingos			

SNACK BARS & SLICES

	QUANTITY	CALS	KJ
Caramel	each	61	258
Chocolate	each	62	263
Raspberry Chocolate	each	61	259
Strawberry Smoothie	each	58	246
NAKED			
Bites			
Cashew & Coconut	each	127	535
Macadamia & Apricot	each	121	507
NATURE VALLEY			
Crunchy			
Apple Crisp	2 bars	188	788
Dark Chocolate	2 bars	195	818
Maple Crunch	2 bars	192	807
Oats & Honey	2 bars	183	799
Roasted Almond	2 bars	199	833
NESTLÉ, MILO Bars	each	107	450
NICE & NATURAL			
Big Nut Chocolate			
Chocolate	each	267	1120
Original	each	265	1110
Yoghurt	each	265	1110
Caramel Nut Bar			
Almond	each	151	633
Original	each	150	628
Chewy Homestyle			
Almond	each	172	723
Apricot	each	164	689
Cranberry	each	159	667
Chocolate Nut Bar			
Almond	each	141	590
Apricot	each	138	580
Original	each	143	600
Fruit Strings			
Blueberry, Raspberry & Strawberry	each	57	241
Raspberry Sours	each	56	235

	QUANTITY	CALS	KJ
Muesli Bars			
Apricot	each	126	528
Chocolate	each	135	565
Yoghurt	each	134	564
Natural Nut Bars			
Apricot	each	158	662
Chocolate	each	163	683
Original	each	150	630
Trail Mix	each	150	630
Yoghurt	each	150	630
Superfruits			
Cranberry & Blueberry	each	109	456
Raspberry & Pomegranate	each	115	481
Strawberry & Blackcurrant	each	121	507
PAMS			
Bubble Bar			
Choc Caramel	each	83	351
Choc Rainbow	each	81	342
Fruity Cereal Bar			
Apple Berry	each	180	757
Superb Strawberry	each	180	755
Tangy Apricot	each	182	764
Muesli Bars			
Apricot	each	119	500
Choc Honey	each	133	560
Oaty Choc	each	124	521
Muffin Bar			
Mango Fruit Snack Bar	each	75	315
Raspberry & White Chocolate	each	148	620
Triple Choc	each	137	575
Oat Bake Bar			
Apricot & Chocolate	each	162	678
Dark Chocolate Chip	each	173	725
Tandem Cereal Bar			
Apple Berry	each	180	757

SNACK BARS & SLICES

	QUANTITY	CALS	KJ
Apricot	each	184	771
Apricot & Custard	each	130	548
Blueberry & Strawberry	each	131	552
Spiced Apple	each	180	757
Strawberry	each	179	753
QUAKER			
Chewy, Apricot	each	101	424
Fibre Bar			
Dark Choc	each	103	434
Wild Berry	each	104	438
Fruit Twists			
Berry Combo	each	126	529
Strawberry Smoothie	each	119	500
Nutbar			
Almond & Berry	each	131	550
Macadamia & Apricot	each	131	550
Mixed Nut	each	133	560
SELECT			
Nut Bar			
Choc & Nut	each	208	868
Macadamia & Cranberry	each	201	844
Rice Bar			
Chocolate	each	90	378
Vanilla	each	92	383
SIGNATURE RANGE			
Fruit Cereal Bars			
Apricot	each	188	789
Mixed Berry	each	188	789
TASTI			
Bars			
Almonds, Cranberries & Apricots	each	136	572
Almonds, Sunflower Seeds & Linseeds	each	142	596
Papaya, Pineapple & Coconut	each	137	575
Fruitsies			
Apple Vanilla	each	70	294

	QUANTITY	CALS	KJ
Strawberry Vanilla	each	70	293
Harvest Bar, Apricot	each	137	575
Mega Nuts Bars			
Caramel	each	213	893
Double Chocolate	each	212	888
Nutty Crunch	each	212	889
Peanut Butter	each	215	902
Milkies			
Choc Strawberry	each	65	276
Choc Vanilla	each	66	279
Muffin Bakes			
Chocolate Fudge	each	144	603
Double White Chocolate	each	144	603
Nut Bars			
Choc Apricot, Coconut & Cashew	each	184	774
Chocolate Almond	each	180	755
Nut Deluxe	each	191	800
Yoghurt, Fruit & Nut	each	170	715
Protein Bars			
Nutty Choc	each	200	835
Roasted Peanut	each	203	851
Salted Caramel	each	196	820
Snak Logs			
Carob Coated Apricot	each	188	787
Carob Coated Fruit & Nut	each	189	792
Oats, Golden Syrup & Coconut	each	167	702
Peanut Brownie	each	179	753
UNCLE TOBYS LeSnak, all flavours	each	83	350
WEIGHT WATCHERS			
Baked Bar			
Apple Strudel	each	84	352
Caramel Shortcake	each	86	363
Chewy Chocolate	each	89	376
Raspberry & White Choc	each	84	354
Cereal Bars			

SNACK BARS & SLICES/SOUP

	QUANTITY	CALS	KJ
Apple Crumble	each	121	508
Apricot Pie	each	121	508
Raspberry Pie	each	135	568
Indulgent Bars			
Coconut Delight	each	89	374
Choc Delight	each	86	361
Nut Bars			
Almond & Apricot	each	151	632
Hazelnut & Orange	each	155	650
Macadamia & Cranberry	each	152	637
Nut Deluxe	each	151	632

Soup

ARTISANO			
Lamb, Israeli Couscous & Mint	100g	48	201
Lentil, Leek & Smokey Bacon	100g	91	382
Hungarian Beef & Paprika	100g	70	296
Pumpkin & Parmesan	100g	41	172
CAMPBELL'S			
Condensed Soups			
Cream of Chicken	per serve	131	549
Cream of Mushroom	per serve	110	464
Cream of Pumpkin	per serve	137	576
Tomato	per serve	79	332
Country Ladle			
Butternut Pumpkin	per serve	108	452
Chicken & Sweet Corn	per serve	114	477
Chicken Noodle	per serve	111	466
Creamy Chicken	per serve	125	527
Farmhouse Vegetable	per serve	81	340
Hearty Beef & Vegetable	per serve	135	568
Minestrone	per serve	96	405
Potato & Leek	per serve	160	670
Rich & Creamy Pumpkin	per serve	118	494

	QUANTITY	CALS	KJ
Roast Chicken & Winter Vegetables	per serve	135	566
CERES ORGANICS			
Mediterranean	per serve	50	212
Tomato & Basil	per serve	80	336
Tuscan-Bean	per serve	86	364
CONTINENTAL			
Cup-A-Soup			
Chicken Noodle	per serve	45	188
Cream of Chicken	per serve	86	360
Cream of Mushroom	per serve	82	342
Pea & Ham	per serve	78	328
Pumpkin	per serve	75	315
Spring Vegetable	per serve	56	234
Tomato	per serve	79	332
Cup-A-Soup Asian			
Chinese Chicken & Corn	per serve	127	532
Laksa	per serve	144	601
Thai Red Curry	per serve	131	550
Cup-A-Soup Croutons			
Creamy Chicken & Corn	per serve	137	571
Creamy Mushroom, Bacon & Sour Cream	per serve	132	552
Creamy Potato & Bacon	per serve	115	480
Creamy Pumpkin	per serve	125	521
Creamy Vegetable	per serve	129	538
Cup-A-Soup Hearty			
Dutch Curry & Rice	per serve	123	514
Italian Minestrone	per serve	145	607
Pea & Ham	per serve	113	472
Roast Chicken	per serve	166	692
Winter Vegetable	per serve	132	551
DELMAINE			
Bacon & Lentil	300g	183	766
Chicken Chowder	300g	146	601
Classic Mushroom	300g	137	575

SOUP

	QUANTITY	CALS	KJ
Red Pepper & Chickpea	300g	198	830
Seafood Chowder	300g	187	786
Traditional Pumpkin	300g	196	821
HANSELLS			
All Natural Soup			
Chicken & Corn	100g	50	208
Miso	100g	63	266
Thai Pumpkin	100g	21	87
Vegetable Tagine	100g	124	521
KING			
Soup Mix, when prepared as directed			
Country Chicken	100mL	34	141
Hearty Vegetable	100mL	35	146
Minestrone	100mL	35	145
Pea & Ham	100mL	33	140
Vegetable	100mL	34	142
MAGGI			
Packet Soups, when prepared as directed			
75 Calorie Sweet Soy & Ginger Chicken	100mL	30	125
Bacon & Onion	100mL	25	95
Chicken Noodle	100mL	10	40
Creamy Chicken	100mL	59	248
Creamy Potato & Leek	100mL	20	85
Creamy Seafood	100mL	25	105
Crème of Chicken	100mL	25	100
French Onion	100mL	15	65
Hearty Oxtail	100mL	25	95
Mushroom	100mL	21	90
Onion	100mL	20	80
Pumpkin & Roasted Garlic	100mL	30	110
Rich Tomato	100mL	25	105
Thick Country Vegetable	100mL	26	110
Soup for a Cup			
Chicken & Sweetcorn	100mL	20	100

	QUANTITY	CALS	KJ
Chicken Noodle	100mL	15	65
Cream of Mushroom	100mL	30	125
Creamy Chicken	100mL	25	110
Creamy Chicken Curry	100mL	25	105
Creamy Chicken Vegetable	100mL	20	95
Golden Pumpkin	100mL	35	150
Hearty Beef & Tomato	100mL	25	115
Rich Tomato	100mL	38	160
Spanish Style Tomato	100mL	37	160
Soup for a Cup, Asian			
Thai Chicken Curry	100mL	38	160
Tom Yum	100mL	38	160
Soup for a Cup with Croutons			
Cream of Chicken & Corn	100mL	51	215
Cream of Tomato	100mL	52	226
Peppered Steak & Mushroom	100mL	52	220
PAMS			
Cup of Soup			
Chicken Noodle	100mL	19	83
Creamy Chicken	100mL	20	86
Creamy Mushroom	100mL	19	82
Farmhouse Pumpkin	100mL	27	117
Rich Tomato	100mL	53	111
Liquid Pouches			
Chicken Chowder	100mL	44	188
Mushroom	100mL	34	146
Pumpkin Soup	100mL	26	112
Seafood Chowder	100mL	47	200
Packet Soup Mix			
Chicken	100mL	33	63
Mushroom	100mL	16	70
Oxtail	100mL	19	83
Seafood	100mL	23	98
Tomato	100mL	23	98
Soup Mix	100g	102	430

SOUP

	QUANTITY	CALS	KJ
PITANGO			
Free Range Chicken Miso	300g	103	434
Free Range Spiced Chicken	300g	300	1257
Organic			
Beef & Lentil	300g	150	630
Broccoli & Blue Cheese	300g	107	449
Chicken Noodle	300g	156	655
Leek & Potato	300g	165	693
Minestrone	300g	114	480
Moroccan Chicken with Mint, Chickpea & Cumin	300g	193	810
Pumpkin with Ginger	300g	94	397
Spring Lamb with Red Wine & Rosemary	300g	174	732
Sweet Potato with Coconut & Ginger	300g	195	817
Thai Pumpkin	300g	117	492
Tomato with Thyme	300g	84	354
Vegetable & Quinoa	300g	114	477
Pea & Ham	300g	219	919
Portobello Mushroom	300g	156	655
Seafood Chowder	300g	138	578
SEASONS			
Kumara, Coconut & Lemongrass	250g	218	915
Pumpkin, Parmesan & Basil	250g	207	868
Smoked Kahawai Chowder	250g	298	1250
Wild Mushroom & Truffle Oil	250g	152	640
SELECT SOUP SACHETS			
Asian			
Laksa	100mL	52	218
Red Curry	100mL	47	197
Croutons			
Chicken & Corn	100mL	49	206
Cream of Chicken	100mL	53	221
Pea & Ham	100mL	42	174
Pumpkin	100mL	44	184
Hearty			

	QUANTITY	CALS	KJ
Dutch Curry & Rice	100mL	45	188
Tomato	100mL	50	209
SIGNATURE RANGE			
Chicken & Corn Chowder	100g	58	244
Creamy Pumpkin	100g	88	372
Creamy Seafood	100g	70	297
Mediterranean Tomato	100g	39	164
TASTY POT			
Chicken & Leek	100mL	45	192
Thai Pumpkin	100mL	42	177
Tomato & Basil	100mL	87	366
THE GOOD TASTE COMPANY			
Cajun Chicken Gumbo	100g	46	195
Creamy Mushroom with Port	100g	43	180
Creamy Pumpkin	100g	63	265
Fish & White Wine Chowder	100g	52	220
Garden Vegetable	100g	52	220
Homestyle Country Chicken	100g	40	170
Kumara & Vegetable	100g	52	220
New York Corn & Bacon Chowder	100g	65	275
Thai Green Buttercup & Coconut	100g	71	300
Tomato & Capsicum	100g	51	215
TRIDENT			
Chicken	100g	44	183
Hot & Spicy	100g	70	294
Tom Yum Goong	100g	148	199
WATTIE'S			
Big 'n Hearty Soup			
Beef Hotpot	100g	40	170
Beef, Vegetable & Barley	100g	47	200
Butter Chicken	100g	89	375
Chicken Gumbo	100g	48	205
Corn & Bacon Chowder	100g	68	285
Irish Stew	100g	43	180
Peppered Steak	100g	58	452

SOUP

	QUANTITY	CALS	KJ
Ravioli with Tomato & Beef	100g	75	315
Salami, Bacon & Pasta	100g	65	275
Condensed Soups			
Creamy Chicken	100g	47	200
Creamy Mushroom	100g	31	130
Creamy Pumpkin	100g	39	165
Minestrone	100g	35	150
Tomato	100g	25	105
Tomato, Extra Rich & Thick	100g	29	125
Tomato, Reduced Salt	100g	25	105
Vegetable	100g	25	105
Soup for One			
Cream of Pumpkin	100g	41	175
Creamy Chicken & Vegetable	100g	38	160
Creamy Tomato	100g	64	270
Tomato	100g	28	120
Vegetables & Beef	100g	46	195
Soup of the Day			
Harvest Pumpkin & Veg	100g	44	185
Minted Garden Pea	100g	35	150
Mushroom	100g	39	165
Thai Style Chicken	100g	66	280
Old Fashioned Chicken	100g	51	215
Spanish Style Chicken	100g	62	260
Spicy Pumpkin	100g	51	215
Vipe Ripened Tomato with Capsicum	100g	38	160
Very Special Soups			
Beef, Vegetable & Pasta	100g	53	150
Chicken & Mushroom	100g	60	255
Chicken & Vegetable	100g	33	140
Chinese Chicken & Corn	100g	58	245
Country Chicken	100g	50	210
Creamy Chicken	100g	60	255
Creamy Corn	100g	47	200
Creamy Mushroom	100g	35	150

	QUANTITY	CALS	KJ
Creamy Pumpkin	100g	53	225
Creamy Tomato	100g	51	215
Italian Minestrone	100g	40	170
Kumara & Vegetable	100g	51	215
Moroccan Bean	100g	65	275
Pea & Ham	100g	52	220
Potato & Leek	100g	40	170
Pumpkin & Vegetable	100g	50	210
Spicy Winter Vegetable	100g	35	150
Thai Spicy Pumpkin	100g	63	265
Tomato & Basil	100g	43	180
Tomato & Capsicum	100g	44	185
Vegetable & Barley	100g	48	205

Spreads

3 BEES			
Creamed Honey	100g	334	1401
Honey	100g	325	1360
100% NUTZ			
Chocolate Peanut Spread	100g	592	2480
Crunchy, Natural	100g	616	2578
Crunchy with Sea Salt	100g	616	2578
AIRBORNE			
Clover	100g	325	1360
Manuka	100g	325	1360
Vipers Bugloss	100g	325	1360
ANATHOTH			
Breakfast Marmalade	100g	270	1130
Jams			
Apricot	100g	272	1140
Blackberry	100g	279	1170
Blackcurrant	100g	277	1160
Boysenberry	100g	274	1150
Cherry Berry	100g	270	1130

SPREADS

	QUANTITY	CALS	KJ
Plum	100g	270	1130
Raspberry	100g	277	1160
Rhubarb & Red Berry	100g	267	1120
Strawberry	100g	270	1130
Three Berry	100g	272	1140
Lemon Curd	100g	325	1360
Marmalade with Ginger	100g	268	1120
Quince Conserve	100g	263	1100
Seville Orange Marmalade	100g	268	1120
ARATAKI, Honey, Manuka & Clover	100g	339	1420
BARKER'S			
Curds			
Lemon	10g	33	139
Lime	10g	31	130
Passionfruit	10g	29	124
Jams			
Apricot	10g	27	113
Black Doris Plum	10g	26	112
Blackcurrant	10g	26	112
Cherry Morello	10g	27	115
Raspberry	10g	27	113
Seedless, Blackberry	10g	26	112
Strawberry	10g	26	111
Marmalades			
Grapefruit & Orange	10g	26	112
Lemon & Lime	10g	27	113
Mandarin & Ginger	10g	25	108
BOVRIL	100g	152	644
BUDGET			
Clover Blend Honey	100g	289	1210
Multi Flora Honey	100g	325	1360
CERES ORGANICS			
ABC Butter	15g	88	372
Almond Butter	15g	86	362
Almond Peanut Butter	15g	76	321

	QUANTITY	CALS	KJ
Cashew Butter	15g	86	361
Energy Spread	15g	88	371
Peanut Butter, Crunchy	15g	85	357
Peanut Butter, Crunchy, No Salt	15g	88	369
Peanut Butter, Smooth	15g	85	357
Peanut Butter, Smooth, No Salt	15g	88	369
Sunflower Butter	15g	86	360
CRAIG'S			
Jams			
Apricot	100g	272	1140
Apricot, Lite	100g	179	750
Black Doris Plum	100g	262	1100
Blackberry	100g	274	1150
Blackcurrant	100g	262	1100
Blueberry	100g	272	1140
Boysenberry	100g	270	1130
Raspberry	100g	262	1100
Red Plum	100g	262	1100
Strawberry	100g	270	1130
Strawberry, Lite	100g	186	807
Marmalades			
Bitter	100g	265	1110
Breakfast	100g	262	1100
English Style	100g	270	1130
Ginger	100g	274	1150
Sweet Tangelo Orange	100g	267	1120
ETA			
Peanut Butter			
Crunchy	100g	609	2550
Crunchy, No Added Salt	100g	604	2530
Roasted, Heavenly Smooth	100g	607	2540
Smooth	100g	609	2550
Smooth, No Added Salt	100g	604	2530
FERRERO, Nutella	100g	518	2170
FREEDOM FOODS, Vege Spread	5g	8	37

SPREADS

	QUANTITY	CALS	KJ
HEALTHERIES			
Dietex Preserves			
Apricot	10g	22	94
Marmalade	10g	23	98
Strawberry	10g	24	103
HILLARY FOODS			
Peanut	40g	228	956
Peanut & Honey	40g	225	943
HOLLANDS			
Premium Manuka Blend	100g	334	1401
Premium White Clover	100g	334	1401
Rich Native Bush	100g	334	1401
HOMEBRAND			
Breakfast Marmalade	100g	274	1146
Choc Hazelnut	100g	564	2360
Jams			
Apricot	100g	270	1129
Mixed Fruit	100g	271	1132
Plum	100g	272	1135
Raspberry	100g	271	1134
Strawberry	100g	268	1121
Peanut Butter			
Crunchy	100g	615	2570
Smooth	100g	629	2630
JOK'N'AL			
Grape Jelly	15g	11	46
Jam			
Apricot	15g	8	37
Blackberry & Apple	15g	9	38
Blackcurrant	15g	10	42
Blueberry	15g	10	42
Pineapple	15g	9	38
Plum	15g	10	41
Raspberry	15g	7	33
Strawberry	15g	8	34

	QUANTITY	CALS	KJ
Lemon Curd	15g	7	29
Orange Marmalade	15g	10	43
KRAFT			
Cheese Spread, Cheddar	100g	277	1160
Original	100g	293	1230
Peanut Butter			
Crunchy	100g	647	2710
Light Crunchy	100g	549	2300
Light Smooth	100g	552	2310
Smooth	100g	635	2670
Vegemite, Original	100g	190	798
Whipped	100g	619	2590
MASTERFOODS, Promite	100g	200	840
OUR MATE, Yeast Spread	100g	231	983
PAMS			
Hazelnut Spread			
Crunchy	100g	580	2430
Smooth	100g	676	2830
Twist	100g	573	2400
Honey, all varieties	100g	325	1360
Jams			
Apricot	100g	270	1130
Apricot & Ginger	100g	272	1140
Blackcurrant	100g	279	1170
Boysenberry	100g	272	1140
Four Fruits	100g	272	1140
Raspberry	100g	267	1120
Strawberry & Rhubarb	100g	270	1130
Marmalades			
3 Fruits	100g	272	1140
Breakfast Grapefruit	100g	270	1130
Chunky Grapefruit	100g	272	1140
Peanut Butter			
Crunchy	100g	607	2540
Crunchy, no added salt	100g	607	2540

SPREADS

	QUANTITY	CALS	KJ
Extra Crunchy	100g	607	2540
Smooth, no added salt	100g	616	2580
PIC'S			
Peanut Butter			
Crunchy, No Salt	100g	568	2380
Original	100g	657	2750
Smooth	100g	568	2380
RED SEAL, Manuka Honey UMF 5+	100g	236	1410
ROSE'S			
Conserves			
Apricot	100g	279	1170
Blackberry	100g	282	1180
Raspberry	100g	272	1140
Strawberry	100g	277	1160
Marmalades			
English Breakfast	100g	274	1150
Ginger	100g	277	1160
Lime	100g	289	1210
Sweet Orange	100g	270	1130
SABATO			
Marmalades			
Sicilian Lemon	20g	46	193
Sicilian Orange	20g	50	211
SANITARIUM			
Marmite	5g	8	25
Peanut Butter			
Crunchy	20g	123	518
Crunchy, No Added Salt or Sugar	20g	121	510
Smooth	20g	123	518
Smooth, No Added Salt or Sugar	20g	121	510
SELECT			
Choc & Caramel	100g	560	2340
Hazelnut	100g	544	2280
Peanut Butter, American Style			
Crunchy	100g	624	2610

	QUANTITY	CALS	KJ
Smooth	100g	631	2640
Peanut Butter			
Crunchy	100g	657	2750
Crunchy, Lite	100g	589	2460
Smooth	100g	634	2650
Smooth, Lite	100g	581	2430
Strawberry & Vanilla	100g	550	2300
SIGNATURE RANGE			
Creamy Honey	100g	325	1360
Liquid Honey	100g	325	1360
Manuka Honey	100g	325	1360
ST. DALFOUR			
Black Cherry	100g	208	870
Blackberry	100g	208	870
Cranberry with Blueberry	20g	208	870
Strawberry	100g	208	870
Thick Apricot	20g	208	870
Thick Cut Orange	20g	208	870
TE HORO			
Apricot	100g	279	1170
Blackberry	100g	305	1280
Raspberry	100g	301	1260
Strawberry	100g	301	1260
WEIGHT WATCHERS, Apricot Fruit Spread	100g	133	560

Tinned Fish

BRUNSWICK			
Tinned Sardines			
Louisiana Hot Sauce	106g	130	543
Mustard Sauce	106g	140	585
Olive Oil	106g	250	1046
Spring Water	84g	130	543
Spring Water, No Added Salt	84g	130	543

TINNED FISH

	QUANTITY	CALS	KJ
Tomato Sauce	106g	140	585
With Hot Peppers	106g	250	1046
DELMAINE, Anchovy Fillets	5g	9	38
GREENSEAS			
Tuna, 98% Fat Free			
Lemon Pepper	100g	139	480
Spicy Chilli	100g	95	400
Sundried Tomato & Basil	100g	143	600
Sundried Tomato & Onion	100g	99	415
Sweet Chilli	100g	169	710
HOMEBRAND			
Mackerel			
In Oil	100g	112	468
In Tomato Sauce	100g	112	468
Sardines			
In Oil	100g	280	1170
In Springwater	100g	210	879
In Tomato Sauce	100g	168	703
Tuna			
Chunks in Brine	100g	95	398
Chunks in Oil	100g	131	552
Chunks in Springwater	100g	105	443
Flaked, Thai Red Curry	100g	136	570
Lemon & Black Pepper	100g	167	702
Light, in Olive Oil	100g	106	444
Smoked	100g	151	632
Sweet Chilli	100g	100	420
Tomato & Onion	100g	158	663
JOHN WEST			
Mussels, Smoked, In Oil	100g	220	923
Oysters, Smoked, In Oil	100g	250	1050
Salmon Slices in Springwater	100g	106	446
Salmon Tempters			
Lemon & Cracked Pepper	100g	148	622
In Springwater	100g	53	225

	QUANTITY	CALS	KJ
Olive Oil	100g	179	752
Onion & Tomato	100g	143	602
Smoked Flavour	100g	121	508
Sweet Chilli & Lime	100g	106	444
Sardine Tempters			
In Oil	100g	262	1100
In Springwater	100g	226	946
In Tomato Sauce	100g	137	576
Tinned Salmon			
Pink	100g	151	634
Pink, No Added Salt	100g	151	634
Red	100g	165	692
Tuna Tempter			
Chunky, in Springwater	100g	113	474
Lemon & Cracked Pepper	100g	92	387
Mango Chilli	100g	129	543
Milk Indian Curry	100g	124	519
Onion & Tomato Savoury Sauce	100g	118	494
Smoked	100g	140	588
Sweet Chilli	100g	92	389
Sweet Seeded Mustard	100g	180	754
Sweetcorn & Mayonnaise	100g	119	498
Tomato Salsa	100g	147	619
Zesty Vinaigrette	100g	142	595
KING OSCAR			
Sardines			
In Olive Oil	85g	240	1004
In Soya Oil	85g	260	1087
Tuna & Beans, Roast Capsium & 3 Beans	100g	155	649
PAMS			
Tinned Mackerel			
In Natural Oil	100g	145	609
In Tomato Sauce	100g	82	345
Tinned Salmon			
Pink	100g	120	505

TINNED FISH

	QUANTITY	CALS	KJ
Pink, Smoked	100g	136	570
Red	100g	165	691
Tinned Tuna			
Lemon Pepper	100g	157	659
Smoked	100g	119	502
Sweet Thai Chilli	100g	160	670
Tomato & Basil	100g	98	414
SEALORD			
Crab Meat	100g	69	289
Fish Fillets, Smoked Flavour	100g	150	628
Peeled Cocktail Shrimps	100g	69	289
Salmon			
Pink	100g	136	570
Pink, No Added Salt	100g	136	570
Pink, Smoked	100g	136	570
Red	100g	163	683
Salmon Sensations			
Cracked Pepper & Lemon	100g	182	764
Light Chilli	100g	187	783
Seeded Mustard	100g	141	594
Smoked	100g	189	791
Spicy Thai	100g	170	714
Sundried Tomato	100g	117	491
Tuna			
In Brine	100g	121	508
In Oil	100g	162	680
In Spring Water	100g	116	488
Tuna, Lite			
Lemon & Cracked Pepper	100g	85	356
Lightly Smoked	100g	87	368
Red Pepper & Chilli	100g	85	388
Sundried Tomato & Basil	100g	90	378
Tuna Sensations			
Lemon Pepper	100g	289	1210
Savoury Onion	100g	117	490

	QUANTITY	CALS	KJ
Smoked	100g	262	1100
Sundried Tomato & Olive	100g	107	451
Sweet Thai Chilli	100g	106	447
Tomato & Basil	100g	121	510
SELECT			
Flaked Tuna			
Lemon & Cracked Pepper	100g	150	631
Lightly Smoked	100g	159	669
Sweet Chilli Sauce	100g	141	590
Tomato Salsa	100g	146	612
Tomato with Basil	100g	125	523
Pink Salmon	100g	120	505
Red Salmon	100g	142	597
Sandwich Tuna in Olive Oil	100g	191	800
Tuna Chunks			
In Brine	100g	109	460
In Extra Virgin Olive Oil	100g	191	800
In Springwater	100g	109	460
TAHI, Mackerel in Oil	100g	142	595
TRIDENT			
Smoked Mussels	100g	349	1460
Smoked Oysters	100g	305	1280
WEIGHT WATCHERS, Tuna in Spring Water	100g	109	460

Tinned Food

	QUANTITY	CALS	KJ
BUDGET			
Baked Beans	100g	83	351
Spaghetti	100g	80	335
CERES, Baked Beans in Tomato Sauce	100g	82	347
DELMAINE, Baked Beans	100g	88	372
HEINZ, Baked Beans	100g	91	385
HOMEBRAND			
Baked Beans	100g	85	357

TINNED FOOD

	QUANTITY	CALS	KJ
Corned Beef	100g	241	1010
Spaghetti	100g	65	275
OAK			
Baked Beans			
In BBQ Sauce	100g	115	485
In Ham Sauce	100g	108	455
In Tomato Sauce	100g	92	385
Spaghetti	100g	54	230
ORGRAN, Spaghetti	100g	62	263
PAMS			
Baked Beans with Sausages	100g	106	445
Spaghetti			
In Tomato Sauce	100g	53	225
With Cheese	100g	59	250
SALISBURY			
Corned Beef	100g	248	1040
Corned Beef, Lite	100g	199	835
Corned Lamb	100g	262	1100
Corned Mutton	100g	270	1132
SELECT			
Baked Beans	100g	93	387
Chicken			
In Brine	100g	132	550
In Springwater	100g	86	358
Mayonnaise	100g	135	563
Mustard & Mayonnaise	100g	144	602
Smoked	100g	83	346
Sweet Chilli	100g	186	776
Tomato & Onion	100g	157	655
Spaghetti	100g	70	292
WATTIE'S			
Baked Beans			
In Tomato Sauce	100g	105	440
Lite	100g	81	340
With Bacon	100g	107	450

	TINNED FOOD/TINNED FRUIT		
	QUANTITY	CALS	KJ
With Meatballs	100g	129	540
With Sausages	100g	119	540
Bean There			
Boston	100g	105	440
Mexican	100g	86	360
Spaghetti			
Cheesy	100g	70	295
In Tomato Sauce	100g	60	255
Lite	100g	64	270
With Meatballs	100g	97	410
With Sausages	100g	86	360
WEIGHT WATCHERS, Baked Beans	100g	86	360
WHOLE EARTH, Organic Baked Beans	100g	103	434

Tinned Fruit

BUDGET			
Apricot Halves In Syrup	100g	71	300
Fruit Salad In Light Syrup	100g	71	301
Peach Slices In Light Syrup	100g	61	258
Pear Halves In Syrup	100g	59	250
Pineapple, Crushed, In Natural Juice	100g	45	192
Pineapple Pieces In Syrup	100g	59	250
Pineapple Slices In Syrup	100g	59	250
CERES ORGANICS			
Apricot Halves	100g	63	264
Peach Slices	100g	54	226
Pear Slices	100g	56	238
Pineapple	100g	49	209
Tropical Fruit Salad	100g	56	238
CINDERELLA			
Sliced Mango, In Light Syrup	100g	69	292
DELISH			
Apple & Cinnamon Pie Filling	100g	81	341
Apple & Mixed Berry Pie Filling	100g	46	195

TINNED FRUIT

	QUANTITY	CALS	KJ
Apple Pie Filling	100g	81	340
Whole Strawberries In Light Syrup	100g	62	260
DELMAINE			
Baby Pears	100g	61	258
Pitted Cherries	100g	71	301
Whole Figs	100g	75	315
DOLE			
Fruit Mix			
In Juice	100g	47	195
In Syrup	100g	86	360
Pineapple Chunks In Juice	100g	62	216
Pineapple, Crushed			
In Juice	100g	62	261
In Syrup	100g	88	368
Pineapple Slices			
In Juice	100g	55	225
In Syrup	100g	86	359
Tropical Fruit Chunks	100g	76	318
Tropical Gold Pineapple			
Chunks	100g	65	272
Slices	100g	65	272
GOLDEN CIRCLE			
Fruit Salad			
Chunky In Natural Juice	100g	56	235
Traditional In Natural Juice	100g	56	235
Traditional In Syrup	100g	82	345
Pineapple			
Pieces In Natural Juice	100g	57	240
Pieces In Syrup	100g	80	335
Slices In Natural Juice	100g	57	240
Slices In Syrup	100g	64	270
GOLDEN SUN			
Apple Pieces In Syrup	100g	71	299
Lychees In Syrup	100g	26	256

	QUANTITY	CALS	KJ
Mango Slices In Syrup	100g	17	73
HOMEBRAND			
Apricot Halves In Syrup	100g	71	298
Fruit Salad In Natural Juice	100g	43	180
Fruit Salad In Syrup	100g	62	260
Peach Slices In Natural Juice	100g	54	230
Peach Slices In Syrup	100g	69	289
Pear Halves In Syrup	100g	68	288
Pineapple			
Crushed In Natural Juice	100g	51	214
Pieces In Natural Juice	100g	45	189
Slices In Natural Juice	100g	41	189
OAK			
Apricot Halves In Light Syrup	100g	69	290
Fruit Salad In Syrup	100g	57	240
Peach Slices In Syrup	100g	76	320
Pear Halves In Syrup	100g	60	255
PAMS			
Crushed Pineapple In Juice	100g	56	237
Crushed Pineapple In Syrup	100g	87	367
Fruit Salad In Juice	100g	57	241
Fruit Salad In Syrup	100g	76	322
Halved Apricots In Juice	100g	48	202
Halved Apricots In Syrup	100g	59	248
Halved Guavas In Syrup	100g	86	360
Mango Slices In Syrup	100g	69	290
Peach Halves In Syrup	100g	69	289
Pear Halves In Syrup	100g	58	245
Pear Quarters In Syrup	100g	58	245
Pineapple Pieces In Juice	100g	54	229
Pineapple Pieces In Syrup	100g	86	361
Pineapple Slices In Juice	100g	54	229
Pineapple Slices In Syrup	100g	86	361
Sliced Apple	100g	54	226
Sliced Peaches In Juice	100g	54	230

TINNED FRUIT

	QUANTITY	CALS	KJ
Sliced Peaches In Syrup	100g	69	289
Whole Black Doris Plums In Syrup	100g	83	350
Whole Blueberries In Syrup	100g	92	385
Whole Boysenberries In Syrup	100g	76	320
Whole Raspberries In Syrup	100g	92	389
Whole Segment Mandarins In Syrup	100g	63	265
Whole Strawberries In Light Syrup	100g	61	256
SELECT			
Apple Sliced	100g	42	177
Apricot Halves In Fruit Juice	100g	48	202
Blackberries In Syrup	100g	103	431
Black Cherries	100g	95	401
Blueberries	100g	92	387
Boysenberries In Syrup	100g	93	387
Fruit Salad In Fruit Juice	100g	54	230
Mango Slices In Syrup	100g	72	301
Mixed Berries In Syrup	100g	80	335
Peach Slices In Syrup	100g	69	288
Pear Quarters In Juice	100g	69	288
Raspberries In Syrup	100g	96	403
SILVERLEAF, Guava Halves In Syrup	100g	69	288
SPC			
Halved Apricots In Juice	100g	66	277
Halved Pears In Lite Juice	100g	47	198
Sliced Peaches In Lite Juice	100g	45	190
TRIDENT			
Lychees In Syrup	100g	87	366
Sliced Mango In Light Syrup	100g	75	315
WATTIE'S			
Apples Sliced	100g	35	155
Apricot Halves In Clear Juice	100g	45	190
Black Doris Plums In Syrup	100g	84	355
Boysenberries In Syrup	100g	77	325
Fruit Salad			
In Clear Fruit Juice	100g	46	195

	QUANTITY	CALS	KJ
In Light Syrup	100g	56	235
Lite, No Added Sugar	100g	26	110
Tropical In Fruit Juice	100g	65	275
Tropical In Light Syrup	100g	65	275
Mango Slices In Light Syrup	100g	68	285
Peach Slices			
In Clear Fruit Juice	100g	41	175
In Light Syrup	100g	46	195
Pear Quarters			
In Clear Fruit Juice	100g	53	225
In Light Syrup	100g	57	240
Lite, With No Added Sugar	100g	33	140
WEIGHT WATCHERS			
Fruit Salad	100g	26	110
Sliced Peaches	100g	20	85

Tinned Vegetables & Legumes

BATCHELORS Peas, mushy	100g	76	323
BUDGET			
Asparagus Pieces In Brine	100g	19	80
Sweet Corn			
Cream Style	100g	70	293
Whole Kernel	100g	84	355
Tomatoes			
Chopped In Juice	100g	16	71
Whole Peeled In Juice	100g	16	71
CERES ORGANICS			
Adzuki Beans	100g	114	480
Black Beans	100g	100	419
Borlotti Beans	100g	86	362
Brown Lentils	100g	76	322
Butter Beans	100g	90	379
Cannellini Beans	100g	116	486
Chickpeas	100g	92	386

TINNED VEGETABLES & LEGUMES

	QUANTITY	CALS	KJ
Chilli Beans, Mild Sauce	100g	92	386
Chopped Tomatoes	100g	19	83
Mixed Beans	100g	84	355
Pinto Beans	100g	92	386
Pomodoro & Basilico (Chopped Tomatoes in Basil)	100g	21	89
Red Kidney Beans	100g	92	386
Refried Black Beans	100g	69	290
Refried Pinto Beans	100g	76	322
Salad Beans	100g	92	386
Soybeans	100g	107	451
Whole Peeled Tomatoes	100g	19	83
CRAIG'S			
Beans			
Cannellini	100g	90	380
Chilli	100g	109	460
Four Bean Mix	100g	112	470
Mexican-style Chilli	100g	103	435
Mixed Bean Salad	100g	95	400
Red Kidney	100g	119	500
Chickpeas	100g	137	575
DELMAINE			
Artichoke Hearts	100g	28	118
Black Beans in Chilli Sauce	100g	87	367
Butter Beans	100g	68	288
Butter Beans in Italian Sauce	100g	85	356
Cannellini Beans	100g	67	282
Chickpeas	100g	81	343
Chickpeas in Curry Sauce	100g	110	461
Chilli Beans	100g	89	373
Four Bean Mix	100g	62	261
Lentils	100g	98	411
Lentils in Curry Sauce	100g	95	400
Passata	100g	12	51
Passata with Basil	100g	35	150

	QUANTITY	CALS	KJ
Ratatouille	100g	43	182
Red Kidney Beans	100g	90	379
Tomato Paste	100g	82	345
Tomato Paste, Double Concentrate	100g	109	460
Tomatoes			
Cherry	100g	25	106
Diced with Chilli, Basil & Oregano	100g	18	77
Diced with Diced Capsicum	100g	20	85
Diced with Fresh Basil	100g	22	93
Diced with Fresh Garlic & Olive Oil	100g	32	135
Italian Crushed	100g	21	92
Italian Diced	100g	21	92
Whole Peeled Roma	100g	23	100
Whole Peeled with Chilli	100g	18	77
With Sliced Olives	100g	51	216
EDGELL, Tiny Taters	100g	68	287
GOLDEN CIRCLE			
Beetroot			
Sliced	100g	59	250
Whole Baby	100g	59	250
GOLDEN SUN, Cut Baby Corn	100g	12	51
HOMEBRAND			
Asparagus Spears	100g	16	68
Corn			
Baby Spears	100g	27	113
Kernels	100g	72	299
Sliced Beetroot	100g	44	186
Tomatoes			
Diced	100g	19	80
Whole Peeled In Juice	100g	19	80
Whole Potatoes	100g	50	213
LEGGO'S			
Pizza Sauce with Garlic, Onion & Herbs	100g	52	221
Tomato Paste			
Garlic & Herbs	100g	55	232

TINNED VEGETABLES & LEGUMES

	QUANTITY	CALS	KJ
No Added Salt	100g	65	275
Original	100g	68	287
Tomato Puree			
No Added Salt	100g	28	118
Original	100g	27	116
MUTTI			
Doppio Concentrato di Pomodoro	100g	96	407
Spicy Pizza Sauce	100g	40	169
Tomatoes, Polpa	100g	26	110
OAK			
Asparagus Spears	100g	21	90
Beetroot Slices	100g	54	230
Chopped Tomatoes	100g	16	70
Creamy Style Corn	100g	87	365
Garden Peas	100g	77	325
OLD EL PASO			
Beans, Refried	100g	76	318
Jalapeños	100g	14	62
PAMS			
Beetroot Slices	100g	54	230
Cannellini Beans	100g	87	366
Chickpeas	100g	120	506
Corn			
Cream Style	100g	86	361
Whole Baby	100g	25	105
Whole Kernel	100g	106	444
Diced Tomatoes			
Basil & Oregano	100g	29	125
Capsicum & Onion	100g	28	121
Chilli & Herb	100g	24	101
Garlic & Oregano	100g	29	125
Whole Peeled	100g	30	128
Red Kidney Beans	100g	102	428
Sliced Mushrooms	100g	25	107
Tomato Purée	100g	40	170

	QUANTITY	CALS	KJ
SABATO, Cherry Tomatoes in Tomato Juice	100mL	20	87
SELECT			
Asparagus Spears	100g	20	83
Beetroot, Sliced	100g	55	230
Borlotti Beans	100g	95	401
Butter Beans	100g	104	436
Chickpeas	100g	117	490
Corn			
Creamed Kernels	100g	56	235
Sweet Kernels	100g	56	235
Five Bean Mix	100g	103	433
Garden Peas	100g	73	306
Lentils	100g	90	378
Lentils, No Added Salt	100g	90	378
Mexican Chilli Beans	100g	114	481
Peas & Carrots	100g	57	241
Peas & Corn	100g	76	321
Red Kidney Beans	100g	101	426
Sliced Beetroot	100g	55	230
Sliced Green Beans	100g	20	129
Tomatoes			
Diced Italian	100g	19	80
Diced Italian, Basil & Garlic	100g	21	90
Diced Italian, Basil & Herbs	100g	21	90
Diced Italian, Basil & Oregano	100g	20	85
Diced Italian, Basil, Garlic & Onion	100g	19	82
Diced Italian, No Added Salt	100g	19	80
Whole Peeled Italian	100g	22	95
WATTIE'S			
Beetroot			
Baby	100g	76	320
Sliced	100g	66	280
Sliced, No Added Salt	100g	64	270
Chickpeas	100g	161	675

TINNED VEGETABLES & LEGUMES

	QUANTITY	CALS	KJ
Chilli Beans			
Hot	100g	103	435
Medium	100g	88	370
Mild	100g	108	455
Corn			
Baby Corn Cuts	100g	22	95
Cream Style	100g	93	390
Cream Style, No Added Sugar	100g	83	350
Whole Kernel	100g	86	360
Whole Kernel, No Added Salt	100g	86	360
Whole Kernel, Organic	100g	86	360
Four Bean Mix	100g	164	690
Green Beans, Sliced	100g	25	105
Indian Style Lentils	100g	64	270
Italian Style Cannellini Beans	100g	90	380
Mexican Style Red Kidney Beans	100g	88	370
Moroccan Style Chickpeas	100g	81	340
Mushrooms			
Sliced in Butter Sauce	100g	38	160
Sliced in Pepper Sauce	100g	86	360
Peas, Minted	100g	113	475
Red Kidney Beans	100g	70	295
Tomato Paste	100g	59	250
Tomato Purée			
Original	100g	40	170
With Herbs	100g	41	175
Tomatoes			
Chopped In Juice	100g	16	70
Chopped In Purée	100g	21	90
Indian Style	100g	46	195
Italian Style	100g	22	95
Moroccan Style	100g	32	135
Pesto Style	100g	37	155
Roast Garlic & Onion	100g	25	105
Savoury	100g	22	95

	QUANTITY	CALS	KJ
Whole Peeled In Juice	100g	17	75
Whole Peeled No Added Salt	100g	17	75

Vegetables & Legumes

Artichoke	100g	27	114
Asparagus, *steamed*	100g	25	103
Baby Sweetcorn	100g	23	95
Beans			
Broad, *boiled*	100g	58	242
Butter, *boiled*	100g	19	81
French (Runner)	100g	17	70
Green, *boiled*	100g	19	79
Mung (Dhal), *raw*	100g	23	95
Red Kidney, *boiled*	100g	102	422
Beetroot	100g	50	207
Broccoli, *raw*	100g	32	134
Brussels Sprout	100g	21	88
Cabbage			
Chinese, *boiled*	100g	12	50
Red, *raw*	100g	23	96
White, *raw*	100g	31	129
Capsicum			
Green	100g	16	66
Red	100g	35	146
Carrot			
boiled	100g	27	112
raw	100g	18	75
Cauliflower, *raw*	100g	27	111
Celery	100g	11	48
Chickpeas, *cooked*	100g	103	429
Chicory	100g	23	96
Chilli	100g	92	386
Chives	1 tsp	0	1
Corn			

VEGETABLES & LEGUMES

	QUANTITY	CALS	KJ
On the Cob	62g	59	245
Whole Kernels	100g	93	385
Courgette (Zucchini)	1 medium	17	72
Cucumber	100g	10	42
Eggplant (Aubergine)	100g	24	100
Endive	100g	17	71
Fennel	100g	31	130
Garlic	per clove	3	12
Gherkin	20g	20	83
Ginger	100g	80	334
Horseradish	100g	36	150
Kale	100g	50	209
Kohlrabi	100g	27	113
Kumara, *baked*	100g	100	413
Leek	100g	28	117
Lentils			
cooked	100g	89	370
split, drained	100g	97	402
Lettuce, *shredded*	1 cup	5	21
Marrow, *boiled, diced*	1 cup	15	68
Mint	25g	18	73
Mushrooms			
raw	1 cup	8	34
fried in butter	1 cup	92	384
fried in oil	1 cup	82	343
Okra	100g	31	130
Onion			
fresh	each	39	161
fried in dripping	1 cup	493	2060
pickled	each	14	58
Rings, breaded	2 rings	81	340
Parsley	1 tbsp	1	4
Parsnip, *boiled*	100g	56	232
Peas			
boiled	100g	78	326

	QUANTITY	CALS	KJ
frozen, boiled	100g	41	171
split, boiled	100g	129	533
Peppers			
Green	100g	26	109
Red	100g	26	109
Pimento	100g	23	96
Plantain	100g	122	510
Potato			
Au Gratin	100g	93	389
baked with skin	100g	88	366
boiled, peeled	100g	87	364
boiled with skin	100g	87	364
Chips, Hot	100g	319	1333
Hash Brown	100g	265	1108
mashed	1 cup	95	394
roasted	100g	105	433
Pumpkin			
baked	100g	46	188
boiled	100g	21	86
roasted	100g	51	214
Radish	100g	19	78
Salsify	100g	68	284
Shallot	100g	70	293
Silverbeet, *boiled*	100g	25	106
Snowpeas	100g	42	176
Spinach, *boiled*	100g	10	41
Spring Onion	100g	32	134
Squash, *steamed*	100g	83	345
Swede, *boiled*	100g	19	79
Taro, *baked*	100g	126	522
Tomato			
chopped	1 cup	32	129
fresh	1 medium	22	86
sundried	1 cup	139	575
Turnip, White, *boiled, mashed*	1 cup	18	74

VEGETABLES & LEGUMES

	QUANTITY	CALS	KJ
Water Chestnuts, *cooked*	100g	97	405
Watercress, *raw*	100g	16	65
Yam, *roasted*	100g	62	257
Dried Vegetables			
Beans, Dried			
Black-eyed	100g	69	289
Butter	100g	94	392
Chickpeas	100g	364	1522
Pinto	100g	347	1450
Red Kidney	100g	85	354
CONTINENTAL, when prepared as directed			
Garden Peas	100g	90	375
Mixed Vegetables	100g	75	315
Peas & Corn	100g	93	390
Sliced Beans	100g	49	205
PAMS			
Pearl Barley	100g	377	1580
Soup Mix	100g	341	1430
Split Red Lentils	100g	296	1240
Split Yellow Peas	100g	325	1360
SUNVALLEY, uncooked			
Brown Lentils	100g	351	1470
Chickpeas	100g	366	1532
Four Bean Mix	100g	343	1436
Green Split Peas	100g	341	1430
Haricot Beans	100g	350	1468
Pearl Barley	100g	351	1470
Red Kidney Beans	100g	333	1394
Red Lentils	100g	351	1470
Soup Mix	100g	346	1450
Yellow Split Peas	100g	341	1430